# What the Health Care Profession Is Saying . . .

"I highly recommend reading this book if you have Arthritis, and I also recommend investigating this product."
— **James P. Carter**, M.D., Dr.P.H., Author, *Racketeering in Medicine, The Suppression of Alternatives.*

"I can't say enough good things about CM Pure™ to which we owe my husband's recovery from 33 years of suffering with osteoarthritis. Now because of the miracle of his healing from debili- tating pain he can take part in physical activities we thought were no longer possible, including swimming and other sports and outings with me and our 3-year-old son. Because CM Pure™ has had such an outstanding effect upon our lives, we feel driven to help improve the quality of everybody's life by sharing it with them. As a result, a number of my patients are now experiencing the same kind of miracles from CM Pure™ that my husband did. I personally believe that CM Pure™ is one of the more potent medical miracles of the century, one that will help heal the suffering of millions with arthritis. Thank you for creating this product."
— **Kathryn Good**, D.C./Q.M.E.

"As a naturopath, I have never seen a product work for arthritis like this one does. It seems to help all forms of Arthritis. I am happy to be a part of this movement that is sweeping the country and getting people well again!"
— **Bruce Lahey**, N.D.

"Centuries of experience of compounding herbs has led the Chinese to develop several unique formulas which are reputed to be effective for the treatment of Arthritis. I find CM Pure™ to be the most effective product yet discovered for Arthritis. I now recommend it to all my Chinese clients."
— Judy Fuse, Ph.D., Pharmacist

"I have found that utilizing nutrition along with chiropractic procedures has helped to build my practice tremendously. We now have a product that will help build your practice as well. This is a product that is ending Arthritis pain for good. I will repeat that statement — for good — in patients with rheumatoid, osteoarthritis and other forms of joint pain."
— Steven D. Moe, D.C.

"As one who has suffered greatly with spinal problems for many years, I have benefitted immensely from CM Pure™ and am pleased to recommend the product to anyone who is suffering from inflammatory pains of any kind."™
— Bob L. Owen, Ph.D., D.Sc.

"All health care professionals at some point come to the realization that you can't always relieve every patient's suffering. Then a product such as CM Pure™ comes along with it's outstanding benefits that can help everyone eliminate the pain of arthritis and other inflammatory conditions. Anybody who has Arthritis or pain associated with tissue inflammation needs to read this book."
— Larry Allen, D.C.

# The Pure Cure for Arthritis

# The
# Pure
# Cure
## for
# Arthritis
## and
## other auto-immune
## and
## inflammatory diseases

Bob L. Owen, Ph.D., D.Sc.

The information in this book is for educational purposes only and is not intended for diagnosing or prescribing. If the reader uses the information to help solve his/her health problems, he/she is prescribing for himself/herself, which is his/her constitutional right, but the author and publisher assume no responsibility.

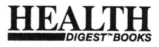

# HEALTH
**DIGEST™ BOOKS**

P.O. Box 1100
Cannon Beach, OR 97110

*The Lord answered me, and said, Write the vision,*
*and engrave it so plainly upon tablets*
*that every one who passes may be able to read it*
*easily and quickly. (Habakkuk 2:2)*

O ye dry bones, hear the word of the Lord,
Thus saith the Lord God unto these
bones; Behold, I will cause breath to enter
into you, and you shall live.
(Ezekiel 37:4-5)

# CONTENTS

# INTRODUCTION

IT ALWAYS SEEMED NATURAL to me that I would become a physician. To begin with, my grandfather was a dentist; my mother a dental hygienist and my father and brother medical doctors. Accordingly, despite a temporary delay of a few years in the military, I proceeded with my inclination and completed my medical education. I have never been sorry for this choice.

Similarly, since my father was a surgeon and I had a gift for working with my hands, it was no problem choosing surgery as my specialty. Although many surgical procedures are not curative, I was impressed that surgery can often more dramatically improve a patient's quality of life than medical therapy.

Doing my surgical residency, I trained under a chief resident (Dr. Maynard Beach) whom I greatly admire and who subsequently became a cardiothoracic surgeon. It was his influence that led me to extend my training in the field of cardiothoracic surgery.

I soon became a busy cardiac surgeon, a very challenging occupation. But over the some 30 years in my profession, I gradually began to recognize many "holes" in the philosophy and practice of orthodox medicine. I saw that in many cases, because of our dependence on the use of drugs, we were not bringing about the curative effects that I believed should be part and parcel of the science of medicine. It seemed to me that something was missing in our armamentarium. Slowly it became increasingly apparent to me that the "missing ingredient" was nutrition.

I began to realize that we (myself in particular, but the profession in general) could be and should be more aggressively including this understanding as part of our therapy to bring about better and longer-lasting patient outcomes.

Still even with this awareness it was difficult at first to effect a change -- or, perhaps more accurately, what I would define as a refinement -- of focus. The reasons were obvious to me. In the first place, nutrition is not taught to any significant extent in medical schools; and, secondly, I, like most of my colleagues, was so busing trying to keep up with my own specialty that I simply had no time even to look at other areas.

I can thank the Price-Pottenger Nutrition Foundation for providing me with a basic understanding of sound principles of nutrition. The name Price-Pottenger comes from two of the early pioneers in the field of nutrition, Dr. Weston Price and Dr. Francis Pottenger. Dr. Price's epidemiological studies and subsequent treatise, *Nutrition and Physical Degeneration*, represent, in my opinion, the most important seminal work in the field of nutrition.

Additionally, Maria, my wife, has greatly enhanced my knowledge of nutrition. Born and raised in the less technologically advanced Ukraine, she and many other Ukrainians have been blessed with much less exposure to prescription drugs and processed foods and therefore have fortunately have had to rely on more whole natural foods and alternative treatments of illness including herbal remedies. especially in such areas as flax seed oil and herbs. Raised in the Ukraine, as she was, along with millions of other so-called "backward" people, she had the advantage of knowing little or nothing of drugs and had to rely upon herbs and good nutrition. Maria is an excellent cook, and makes a wonderful brick-oven baked "Ukrainian black bread" which is sourdough whole grain rye bread made with natural yeast.

Tragically, some of her peoples, as well as others in many parts of the world, have begun to experience deterioration in health as they have accepted more of the modern fabricated processed foods and modern ways of cooking, such as the microwave.

As a cardiothoracic surgeon, I have occasion to speak to my coronary bypass patients about nutrition, which is generally considered to be only a contributing factor by most orthodox physicians. But, unlike many of my colleagues, I believe that coronary artery disease, as well as other degenerative diseases, is not only totally preventable, but can be stopped in its tracks and in most, if not all, cases, even reversed. For this reason I spend a considerable amount of time with my patients trying to educate them how to change their nutritional habits so as to avoid coming back for a second or even a third operation as some of them do.

But it is not an easy task because many of my colleagues are giving them what I consider to be bad nutritional advice and this same bad nutritional advice is being promoted by the food processing industry, the advertising world and even governmental agencies.

Unfortunately, most of my patients are in a critical life-threatening situation by the time I see them and require bypass surgery to prevent a likely imminent fatal heart attack. This is merely a "quick fix" which buys them time to hopefully change their lifestyle to prevent progression of the disease.

Most are very eager but surprised to learn how wrong food choices, including refined carbohydrates, such as white flour and white sugar, "bad" fats and oils and insufficient quality and quantity of fresh fruits and vegetables, combined with certain other lifestyle habits have brought them to the brink of an early demise.

They are shocked to learn how most supermarket foods have been devitalized and stripped of nutrients with "plastic" synthetic additives taking their place. Although many understand that the food processing industry is primarily interested in financial returns, they do not comprehend the extent to which their understanding of nutrition is dominated by commercial interests.

The problem, it seems to me, is simple conceptually. Good food should go bad, in general. But the food processing industry has a major problem with this fact of nature. They have to store their foods in warehouses for periods of time and ship them over long distances. Accordingly, they have to do something to the food to prevent it from deteriorating which means either stripping it of the most nutritious perishable portion of the food, or adding some unnatural additive as a preservative, or both. The unfortunate but inevitable consequence is that long "shelf life" leads to short "people life."

I spend a considerable amount of time lecturing across the nation about the nutritional benefits of whole natural foods; and it was on one such weekend lecture that I met the author of this book, who apprised me of the benefits of the plant-based long-chain fatty acid cetyl ester that he covers so well in the pages that follow.

Although I have no financial interest in this product, based on my understanding of the very important role of fatty acids in the treatment of arthritis, I have every confidence in recommending this to my patients
-- Richard W. Pooley, M.D.

# PROLOGUE

For many years I have believed that arthritis, in its many and varied forms — destructive and crippling though it may be — can be controlled by a rigid, carefully structured lifestyle, including diet. Though not designed by myself, on occasion I have seen such a protocol work.

But, not until Dr. David Allen fortuitously came into my life had I even dared to think that arthritis, instead of merely being controlled, could actually be reversed, even healed or cured. Or, if one prefers to employ euphemistic terminology, put into permanent remission.

It's truly exciting to realize that arthritis is not totally invincible, that this erstwhile crippler has a nemesis. And the nemesis is not an armamentarium of new, exotic and powerful drugs. It is a totally natural compound. The implications of this revelation are staggering!

Does that mean that the men and women, and the children, who are being inconvenienced or handicapped by arthritis in exponentially increasing numbers, can now become free of the disease? The answer is a resounding, Yes!

This miracle is possible because of the discovery and isolation of a previously unknown long-chain fatty acid ester, that was believed to have the capability of preventing arthritis in laboratory animals. However, it was not until two scientists -- Dr. David Allen, nutrition/psychologist and Dr. B.P. Poovaiah, Ph.D., nutrition biochemist -- discovered a way to produce large quantities of a pure, stable, plant-based long-chain fatty acid cetyl ester that the substance could be widely and effectively used.

11

The result is CM Pure™, an advanced biologically active formulation.

CM Pure™ has just now been made easily available to the general public for the first time. And, because this is a natural, non-toxic nutritional supplement, no prescription is needed.

There's never been anything like CM Pure™ before. It's not some sort of pain reliever or anti-inflammatory drug. Derived from a plant source, compatible with human tissue, CM Pure™ is so "user friendly," so beneficial, so unique and precise in its action and — at the same time — so gentle; so effective, that it may well completely revolutionize the way all inflammatory and autoimmune diseases will be treated in the future.

# Chapter One
## THE DIAGNOSIS

Words like *cancer* and *arthritis* have an ominous sound to them. I know they do for me, and I'm quite certain they do for about everyone. I hear them both frequently. I hear those and the names of many other "disease conditions." I don't get used to hearing them. But, that sort of comes with the territory.

In my chosen profession as a nutritional counselor I have the privilege of meeting and dealing with scores of interesting people: many of them vibrant and healthy. Many are somewhat below par and seeking to improve their health. Others are sick and hurting, and attempting to lift themselves — from the edge of the grave itself — by their own bootstraps.

At the moment I can think of a dozen or more who fit that last category. I'd like to think I helped them all to turn both their health, and their lives around. Being realistic, though, I know that's not always the case. Even though you win some; it hurts when you lose others.

But, I do my best. So, with each of those who come to me, I attempt to design a program that will specifically meet the needs of that individual.

Because I know that degenerative diseases must be treated and reversed by both detoxification (to rid the body of an excessive load of toxins and to normalize the acid-alkaline balance), and nutrient enrichment. I know that if total success and regained health is the ultimate goal, neither can be done without the other. Too many try to do one without the other. It's not either/or. It takes both.

When Joe called and asked to see me, I wondered which category he would choose. As I do with them all, I try not to prejudge, because some of them will fool you. Some say they can't, but still do it. Some say they will, but don't. I try to keep an open mind and a positive attitude.

"Who gave you my name?" I asked. I work primarily by referral.

He named a person I know well, who has referred a number of people to me for nutritional counseling. As I do with all who call me, I FAX or mail them a Nutritional Counseling Questionnaire to complete before I'll discuss their concerns with them. Joe's completed questionnaire came back immediately. His answers were pretty straightforward. So we set up a time for a telephone counseling session. The focus of his concern was, "I'm worried about the pains in my back, knees, elbows and arms . . ."

"Arthritis?" I asked bluntly, not wishing to waste either his time or mine.

"That's what the doctor said . . . as he wrote me out a prescription . . ."

It was because of something I heard in his voice — and because of some new research I had become involved in — that I invited Joe to meet me at my condominium office that overlooks San Diego's gorgeous bay. When I saw him, and spent a few minutes talking to him, I realized two things: One, Joe was in much more trouble than he'd admitted to on the phone. And, second, there was something indomitable in his eye and his spirit that refused to be defeated. It was the latter that made me believe he was one of the group that would "make it."

For a few minutes we chatted about sailing, and gloried in the beauty of the Bay that was alive with hundreds of sailboats.

"Before I can be of any help to you, Joe . . ." I began, "You've got to tell me much, much more about yourself. Don't leave out anything . . ."

Indicating Joe's painful limp and the awkward, uncomfortable way he sat and moved himself about on the deck chair, I continued, "Because, I want to know how you allowed yourself to get into this condition."

Joe nodded and sucked in a deep breath of the fresh salt air.

For the next couple of hours, Joe related a story of suffering and pain that's become all too familiar, far too commonplace to our society as a whole, but especially to most health practitioners. Rather than telling you Joe's story, I'll let you listen in while he shares it with us both in his own words . . .

*****

*I was born in Montana . . .* he began.

*My father owned this big ranch. We raised cattle. And almost from the time I was able to walk, I was put in the saddle. By the time I was in the third or fourth grade I was helping with the Spring roundup. We'd go out into the brush and bring in all the new mothers and their new calves to be branded.*

*I loved it. But it was hard work. Many a day I'd sit saddle for twelve or more hours, and by the time the day was over, I couldn't dismount. I'd actually fall out of the saddle. I'd have a dickens of a time straightening myself out and standing to my feet. Many a night I was so stiff and sore from riding all day long that I couldn't sleep.*

*I did this every year of my life till I went off to college. I guess the hard work and the weather took its toll. In the summer the heat and dust was almost unbearable. In the winter, the snow was deep and we had to go out and feed the cattle. Many of those winter nights my bones ached all night long and the pain in my back and legs kept me awake.*

15

*Because of my size they put me on the football team. I'm over six feet, and weigh two-twenty, or should. Right now I'm about twenty pounds heavier than I'd like to be. Anyway, they put me on the football team.*

*They didn't have to force me. I loved it. I was in good condition: muscles tough and hard, reflexes excellent. I was fast and aggressive. So I gave some rough hits. And I took plenty of them. After a couple of years on the team, I got so stoved up that I could hardly walk.*

*I suppose that was the beginning of my troubles. My knees started popping and cracking when I walked. My back was always stiff, so I could hardly bend it.*

*It was about then that I first began to realize that something was going on in my body that could quite possibly be serious.*

*That was about ten years ago. Ten hellish years.*

*I had been to chiropractors a lot. I'd get thrown from a horse and I had to have my bones straightened out again so I could get back on the horse. I'd even had a few broken bones that had to be set. But, I've been pretty lucky. Up until about ten years ago I'd never been to a doctor, a medical doctor, I mean, for anything other than to get a rib taped up or a cast on my leg. Something like that.*

*But, about ten years ago, eleven, to be exact, I got to hurting so bad that I couldn't stand it. I had taken so many aspirin that my stomach began to bleed, and I got scared. Like I said, I was hurting real bad, so I made an appointment with this doctor. A specialist. An orthopedic surgeon.*

*He was the first one to tell me I had arthritis.*

*"You've got it really bad," he told me. "All through your back and pelvis. Hands, shoulders, knees. Man, you're in a heck of a shape!"*

*I guess he was right. I felt like it. And I hobbled around like a man of eighty. Even though I was only twenty five.*

"What'll I do?" I asked.

He got out his little pad and wrote a prescription. "Get this at the drug store," he told me. "It'll make you feel better."

"Is it going to help cure my arthritis?"

He shook his head. "Man, nothing's going to cure that. About all we can do is try to control the pain."

I hurt so bad and felt so bad, I did something I'd done only a couple of times in my life. I got drunk. I suppose I thought it would help me some. But, it didn't. All I got was a hangover and a bruised hip when I fell down in the bar room. The next morning I was a mess. I hurt all over. I was trying to recover from the tailspin the doctor's words had put me in.

I guess I've never recovered from his words — nothing would cure me. All I had to look forward to was the rest of my life on pain killers. As bad as I felt, I wanted to go out and get drunk again. Maybe it would all go away. I did, that is, got drunk again. But it didn't go away.

And it hasn't for these last eleven years. What a way to live.

Joe and I talked for a couple of hours that first day. By that time his back and hips were hurting so bad that he couldn't sit still. We agreed to meet again in a few days . . .

17

## Chapter Two
## THE DISEASE

**Arthritis:** I'm very familiar with it.

It's undoubtedly the world's most crippling disease condition. That's been true for many years. And the picture hasn't changed much, except to worsen. Even the statistics released by the Arthritis Foundation, whose declared mission it is to support arthritis research and to try and find the cure for arthritis, are not very encouraging. About 50 million Americans suffer from some form of arthritis, an additional 30-40 million people suffer from low back pain (a high percentage of it being arthritis), and millions suffer from arthritic neck pains. *The Arthritis Foundation's latest figures indicate that by the time we reach the age of 50, at least eighty percent of us are destined to develop arthritis.*

This is not a pleasant prospect.

Further, they indicate that one third of our country's entire adult population is already suffering from osteoarthritis, frequently called degenerative joint disease. An additional two and one-half million are afflicted with rheumatoid arthritis, which is a chronic inflammatory condition that seems to affect the entire body. Even children are being stricken with arthritis, with at least 200,000 being affected by the juvenile form of arthritis.

By this time in his continuing struggle to maintain some sort of emotional normalcy, Joe was more or less aware of the nature — and the usual prognosis — of his condition. He hadn't come to me for this type of information. He came to me to see if I, or anybody, could somehow help him turn his situation around.

"It's about to wreck my entire life," he told me the next time we met. "After graduating from college, I met Helen. And, well, we were attracted to each other. Six or eight months later we were married."

"Happily?"

He shrugged. "Reasonably . . . we've had our ups and downs, like most couples. But, now . . ." His words trailed off and he stared off into the distance. I didn't push him. Just waited for him to continue.

"But now . . ." he turned back, his face twisted in a wry grin. "We can't even make love most of the time. Because, I'm hurting so bad . . . I can hardly bear to have her touch me. Anywhere."

It was a common story, tragic none the less.

"For the first few years of our married life, it was wonderful . . ."

Joe told me about his work. He was a computer programmer. Helen, his wife, owned her own beauty salon.

"An evening a week I'd play basketball with the fellow, and Helen would go to her aerobic dancing class. We'd jog together most mornings. Weekends were special. We didn't usually schedule anything, that is, with other people. Those two days were for us . . ."

Joe's voice trailed off again. I waited.

"Then one day — quite suddenly — my left knee began hurting."

He'd been jogging with Helen when it happened. The pain had been so sharp and intense that he stumbled. He sat down on the grass to catch his breath. A few minutes later Helen turned and saw him just sitting there. She jogged back to where he was sitting on the grass clutching his knee.

He'd tried to play it down as nothing, which is what he'd actually thought: that it was nothing to be concerned about.

He told Helen to go on, he'd sprained himself, but he'd be okay. He'd meet her at home. He limped home carefully, sparing the knee as much as possible. By the time he'd taken a hot shower, the pain had almost totally subsided. The next morning his knee was all right. He tested it gently when he slid out of bed. It was okay. No pain. He pressed it gingerly. Just a slight soreness. Nothing like the day before. He was whistling when he went to work.

"Every day that injured knee was on my mind," he told me.

Again he stared off, seemingly at the cruise liner that was coming into the harbor, flags flying. But I knew he wasn't seeing the ship at all.

The next incident took place on the basketball court. He was dribbling when the guard moved in to grab the ball. Instantly Joe pivoted on  his left foot and slid smoothly beneath the man's hands. When he shot, the ball didn't touch the hoop, just swished right through. But, he was suddenly aware of that deep, dull ache again. He tried to ignore it and finished the game. Again, a soak in the steaming shower eased the pain. By the time he'd gotten home it was gone.

"I worried about it all the time," Joe said, turning back from the cruise ship.

"What did you do about it?"

"Nothing, really. I suppose I thought that if I ignored it that it'd go away." He gave the wry grin I was becoming familiar with. "It did, too . . . at least for a while. Quite a while, in fact."

Actually Joe had done something about the problem, he admitted. He told Helen that he'd probably sprained it more that day when they were jogging than he'd thought. "I think I'll stay off my feet for a few days and let it rest."

21

Which he had done. He even stopped playing basketball for a few weeks. At nights he would soak in a tub of hot water. For several weeks he had no pain at all. No twinges, no dull ache. Nothing.

"At first I couldn't believe it. But when a month or so went by, I hoped I'd just imagined the whole thing . . . and I started playing ball again."

"Then what?" I probed.

"Nothing happened. Not for several days. Then it happened at work . . ." As a computer programmer, Joe's work life was quite sedentary, which was part of the reason why he made certain he scheduled some aerobic exercise in his leisure hours.

This time, he was sitting at his computer console, tensely concentrating on an especially challenging task, when it hit him.

"Just like that!" Joe snapped his fingers. "Just like that it hit me. And just like that it was gone." The sudden pain broke his concentration.

"What did you do?"

"Quit early, went home and soaked in the tub."

"And that helped?"

Joe drew a long, deep breath. "For the moment," he told me. "But from then on the pains came more and more closely together. I thought maybe it was because I was thinking about them all the time. Maybe I was causing them to come."

He looked me directly in the eye. "Look, Dr. Bob, is it possible to focus on something so much that you can cause it to happen? Like a sort of unconscious pain wish? Something like that?"

"Of course, Joe, anything's possible. The mind's very powerful. But, if that possibility is true, couldn't just the opposite be just as viable?"

"What do you mean?"

As he spoke, Joe turned so suddenly to face me that I observed that it brought a fresh spasm of pain to his shoulder.

"If the mind could help cause the problem, Joe. Couldn't the mind just as well help bring healing to the problem?"

His answer was thoughtful and slow in coming. "I hadn't thought of that. Is that something like visualization?"

I nodded. "That's what I was thinking. But don't get me wrong, Joe. I'm not trying to say you can just *think* the pain away. Visualization is much, much more than mere *thinking*."

"Then, just what is visualization if it isn't thinking?"

Now it was my turn to answer slowly. "Joe, I don't think you're quite ready for this. Not yet. We've got a lot more ground to cover. And visualization works best when it's combined with a total lifestyle and nutritional program."

As open as Joe appeared, I seemed to feel a hesitancy in him to relate the entire story of his battle. It was as though he felt ashamed of having succumbed to arthritis in the first place; and that he could have, should have, done more for himself than he had. As yet, Joe hadn't asked me for advice. So I hadn't given any. He just seemed to feel an urge to bare his soul to me. I bided my time.

*****

"It's been rough, Dr. Bob," he told me one day. "I think I've done about all there is to do . . . but I get the feeling from Helen that I should be doing more . . ."

"Like more what?"

Joe didn't answer me directly.

He eased himself slightly in his chair and a grimace of pain slid across his forehead that was prematurely wrinkled by the continual assault of pain. After a while, he sighed sadly. "Fortunately, I've got good medical insurance. Or did have. I'm afraid my coverage is about to expire . . ."

23

Joe searched me with his intense eyes, as though seeking permission. "Mind if I tell you a little of what I've gone through?"

"Not at all." I crossed my legs and made myself more comfortable. "Shoot."

*****

*All my life I've been strong . . . he began.*

*Nobody ever had to do anything for me. I've always been self-sufficient and self-willed. Too much so at times. Like now, with this problem . . .*

*Helen's not that way. She's independent too, but different. If she can't do something immediately, she's not too proud to ask for help. So, when she calls for me, I come running. Thing is, though, it's a lopsided arrangement. Even if I could use help, I never ask for it. I grit my teeth and do it myself. Or die trying.*

*When it got difficult for me to get in and out of the car, she offered to drive. I wouldn't let her. I'm the man, I said to myself. And a man takes care of his wife. Not the other way around. At least in things like this. So, at first she let me do it. She could see how much pain I was in, but didn't say much. Finally, one day my pain and discomfort became so evident; and I became so clumsy that I simply could not climb into the driver's seat.*

*Helen didn't say a word. She took my arm and guided me around to the passenger side and helped me in. All the while I was burning with shame and embarrassment. My macho just couldn't take it. Everything hit me at once: My inability to get into the car; to help around the house; to play basketball with the boys; to make love with my wife . . .*

*I just broke down and sobbed. Right there in the car. With her beside me. Again, Helen didn't say a word. She just stroked my hair like she used to when we first met and were first married. Then she bent and kissed my ear and whispered, "Joe, please don't pretend so hard. I know you're*

24

hurting. I know you're trying. But this thing's gotten out of hand. Let's go see a doctor . . . "

I didn't look up. By the time I'd wiped my tears away she had backed out of the driveway and was on the road. I didn't ask any questions about where she was going. But when she drove up in front of a strange office, I had to say something.

"Where are we?"

"We're at the chiropractor's office," she answered in her efficient way. "I called him and made an appointment."

I was in so much pain that I didn't resist when she helped me out of the car and led me into the office like a child, stumbling and unsteady, with her arm around my shoulder. By the time I slumped to a chair, I didn't care where we were. I was all at once besides myself with the whole scene. I was agitated almost beyond my control, but not Helen. She calmly took control of the situation. Before long I was seated in the doctor's office.

Dr. Erikson was a middle-aged man, with a kindly expression. "Well, Joe, talk to me. Tell me what's happening."

Helen sat in the chair next to me holding my hand. She said nothing and let me do the talking. It all came out in a rush. The whole story . . . more than I'd ever told anybody before.

He didn't ask any questions till I'd finished. He just listened.

When I'd finished, he gave me a short cotton gown, told me to put it on, and left the room. To my intense embarrassment and shame, I couldn't undress by myself. Helen had to help me. Very aware of my macho feelings, she made nothing of the incident; she just helped me. And when I was ready, she went to get the doctor, and left me alone with him.

Dr. Erikson's hands were gentle; still I was so tender in many spots that the examination was painful. He didn't really treat me, just checked me over: joints, ligaments, soft muscle tissue, all that. He said very little during the examination. When he was finished, he told me to get dressed, then said he wanted to talk to my wife and me together.

The bottom line was, "I suggest further testing, but preliminarily, it looks like you've developed arthritis in several parts of your body . . ."

"Can you help me?" I blurted out. I was beginning to feel caged in and rather desperate. Helen felt for and squeezed my hand reassuringly.

Dr. Erikson regarded me carefully, as though assessing how much he should tell me; how much of the truth I could handle. He shook his head slowly. "I can possibly help you some. I'm not sure how much. I can probably help relieve some of the pain and discomfort, temporarily. But, that's about the best that you can expect from me, or from any chiropractor . . ."

# Chapter Three
## THE SEARCH

At Joe's insistence, detecting a note of panicky desperation in his voice when he'd called me this morning, I had agreed to meet him at The Vegetarian Zone for lunch. The Vegetarian Zone, one of San Diego's best vegetarian cuisine restaurants, is a favorite of my wife and myself. I ate while Joe talked. He barely sipped his soup. As he shared with me his traumatic experience with the chiropractor, Joe's whole being trembled with emotion. But, it had been just the beginning of his endless — and fruitless — search for relief.

Regarding me now, Joe's face was a mask of pain, only partially controlled by the non-steroidal anti-inflammaatory drugs (NSAIDs) he was taking. I noted the premature gray around his temples, and how he winced as he struggled to handle a soup spoon; his knuckles were taking on the swollen, knobby configuration of the typical arthritic sufferer.

*After leaving the chiropractor's office that afternoon, a cloud of depression seemed to descend upon me and envelop me. There's really no other way that I can describe how I felt that day.*

*Though I am certainly not a quitter, my whole life is a testimony to that fact, I drifted painfully through the next weeks in a blue funk, if that helps paint a picture of how I was. I'm only forty years old, I kept telling myself, and just look at me: I'm fast developing into a cripple.*

*The thought of suicide entered my mind. And I dwelt on that possibility by the hour, for days at a time.*

*The possibility of delivering myself from my prison of pain sounded very attractive, and I considered and finally discarded a number of different modes. Either a particular method would be too gruesome — leaving a macabre mess for someone to clean up, or the execution of it (no pun intended) would require more strength than I could physically manage (such as attempting to hang myself); or the act of firing a bullet into my body required more courage than I could muster; or, the acquisition of the necessary tools of destruction (such as quick-acting poison) would be beyond my capability.*

*Finally, I succumbed to a state of numb semi-existence. I got by, but just barely.*

*Helen tried to lift my spirits in every way she could. She obtained books and pamphlets from the Arthritis Foundation. I looked at them, then tossed them all aside. Perhaps the Foundation's material affects others differently, but the idea of "learning how to live with arthritis," the thread that seemed to pervade all their well intended information, did nothing but drive me more deeply into the abyss into which I had descended.*

*My days were brightened briefly when I came across Norman Cousin's book, **The Anatomy of an Illness,** and I thought he might have keyed into the "cure" for my disease as well as his. This hope was finally shattered for me a bit at a time as I continued to make my rounds of the medical gurus.*

*The acupuncturist helped ease the pain for a few days. Then, all the symptoms returned again with all their force and fury.*

*My visit with the neurologist was disappointing. It seemed that his learned spiel amounted to a complex regurgitation of the Arthritis Foundation's homilies. With the end result the same: learn to live with it. The same was true with the rheumatologist: more drugs, more pats on the back: "Buck up, Buddy . . . you could be worse off, you know."*

*All these non-invasive tests these doctors did, and all the examinations they performed came up with the same answer: "There's nothing organically wrong with your knees. Or any other part of your body."*

*Somehow, these conclusions left me with a growing sense of futility.*

*My next stop was the orthopedic surgeon.*

*In all due respect, all of the professionals I submitted myself to had clearly done the best they could with the means at their disposal. The orthopedist did the same. Her examination was thorough. And painful (as had been all the others). However, there was a difference.*

*Whereas the examinations of all the others had been non-invasive, this doctor suggested arthroscopic surgery. "Xrays and MRIs," she told me, "cannot give a truly accurate picture of what's happening. Let's go in, open up your left knee (the point of the greatest disfigurement and pain) and get a good look."*

*Hoping against hope that she would find something encouraging, I agreed. After all, the insurance was paying for it, wasn't it? Might as well get my money's worth. All cynicism aside, I do appreciate the fact that my insurance did allow me to examine every single option I could locate that was available to me.*

*When it was all over with, she sat me down in her office. As she looked at me kindly and compassionately from across her desk, I couldn't help but note, and read, all the plaques, certificates and awards on the wall behind her. I expectantly awaited her words of wisdom, which weren't long in coming.*

*Instead of speaking immediately, the doctor arose from her desk and moved to an easel that stood in the corner of her office. She opened a flip chart and leafed through a few pages until she came to a page showing two different views of a joint, one above the other.*

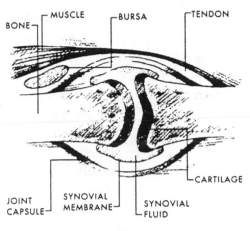

Healthy joint

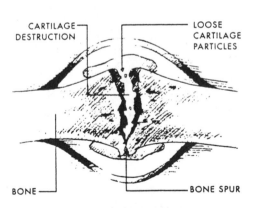

Osteoarthritic Joint
Courtesy the Arthritis Foundation.

**Above: Normal, healthy joint with smooth, well-lubricated cartilage. Below: Pitted and worn away cartilage, a condition that results in pain and possible further damage.**

*As though teaching a class in anatomy — which one of the certificates indicated that she did indeed teach courses in the subject — she used a wooden pointer to show me the upper of the two pictures.*

*"This picture, as you can see, Mr. James, shows a normal joint . . ." As she spoke, she used the pointer to designate joint nomenclature. Moving quickly from one spot to another, she stopped at the center of the joint. "Notice how the ends of each bone is covered with a thick layer of tissue. This is cartilage, designed both for flexibility and to help cushion the shock when you place weight on the bones, and the two ends of the bone come together . . ."*

*I quickly saw that the bone ends in the first picture were cushioned sufficiently. Even before the doctor moved her pointer, my eyes moved to the lower picture. Instantly, I could see the problem. ". . . cartilage in this picture has been damaged. The pain, stiffness, crackling and heat comes from these two damaged bone ends rubbing together, bone on bone. With little or no cartilage to cushion the shock . . ."*

*She tapped the picture of the damaged joint for emphasis. "Look at this."*

*I looked and gasped. I had seen these pictures in some of the brochures I had received, but this doctor had personalized them. Before, I hadn't completely understood them. Now I did. Perfectly. And I didn't like what I saw, or what it seemed to mean.*

*"This could be a picture of your joints," she said. "You have some cartilage degeneration . . ." She paused and allowed the words to sink in, which they did, quickly and deeply. "Perhaps not as bad as this picture. But degenerated enough for you to do everything you can do to prevent it from getting worse."*

*She paused again, then added, "However . . . there is good news."*

"What's that?" I blurted out, grasping at any available straw.

"The cartilage in your joints, isn't completely worn through."

"What does that mean?"

"You've got to begin taking better care of your joints."

"How? What . . . what can I do?"

She shook her head sadly, as others had done. "Your exercise will have to be confined to walking. Regularly. And swimming. But, no jogging, Mr. James. No jogging, or basketball . . ."

"Which I haven't done for months," I said bitterly.

She went on, "Take this medication. Hope for the best. Learn to live with it. Grin and bear it. Sorry, that's the best that can be done."

The best that can be done.

"Dr. Bob," Joe was saying to me, "those words rang in my mind for days. That's the best the medical profession can do for me. The ultimate. The very best."

His shoulders drooped and he slumped in his chair.

I thought it was time to tell Joe, that there just might be something more that can be done, not just to alleviate the pain, swelling and disfigurement of arthritis. But even the possibility of reversing the progress of the disease.

## Chapter Four
## THE CAUSES

    As I carefully studied the joint diagram in the book I held in my hands, once again I marveled at the complexity of our bodies, and how important it is for us to understand the basics of physiology. There are many different types of cartilage in the body, each performing many different functions. But the cartilage found in the joint is *articular* cartilage; which is the magic substance that must be present and healthy for smooth, painless movement in the joints.

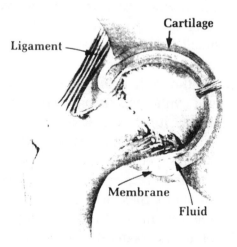

**A normal, healthy hip joint.**

    In the normal course of events, as the cartilage surfaces glide over one another thousands and hundreds of thousands of times, some of the exposed cells die and peel away. This happens on a minute by minute, hour to hour basis. And when the exposed cells are dispatched, new cartilage cells take their place from the growing ends that are attached to the bone surfaces on the two sides.

*That's the normal course of events. But when, for one reason or another, the system fails, arthritis is the result.*

Defined as an inflammation or pain in a joint or joints in any of the human body's 143 different joints — in shoulders, knees, elbows, hips, fingers, back, even the seeming immovable bones of the skull, and more — arthritis probably causes more pain and suffering than any other disease condition.

The causes of arthritis are extremely complex and varied. For the most part, they are not totally understood, and may not be exactly the same from body to body or person to person. They may range from genetics, infection, stress, injury, disease; poor, wrong or inadequate nutrition; dehydration, cumulative wear and tear across the years; or a combination of any or all the above. Considering each of these one at a time, I believe that most degenerative conditions are reversible.

## Genetic and Other Self-Limiting Conditions

Often charged with responsibility for arthritis and other disease conditions, it is true that genetics undoubtedly play a part with some. Certain specific genetic conditions, affecting a total of about 5 per 1,000 individuals, may not be totally curable, but most respond to detoxification and biological nutritional approaches. It is also true that human bodies eventually wear out, most of them many years sooner than they should or could. Natural nutritional approaches have been proven to be effective for reversing or preventing degenerative diseases that result from eating habits and lifestyles out of line with nature.

Stressful living and working environments tend to erode the quality of life and contribute to a gradual breakdown of tissues, resulting in degenerative conditions such as heart and circulatory disease, cancer, diabetes and arthritis. The same applies to infections, injuries and cumulative dehydration. All produce chemical and physiological changes in cells, tissue and organs that result in disintegration and breakdown, often resulting in trauma to joints and cartilage. *A condition we know as arthritis.*

Coupled with any or all other causes, most scientists and health practitioners agree, that over time, poor or inadequate nutrition plays a significant role in either the health or degeneration of the entire bone complex.

### Degenerative Conditions Are Reversible

Whatever the cause, *degenerative conditions are reversible*, which is not always the case with degenerative diseases. Because, there is a point of no return that happens when vital organs have been damaged beyond their ability to function or to recover. Nobody knows when that point has been reached, which is different for every person. For that reason alone, if for no other, nobody should give up and quit trying to improve his or her health. And no health professional should "write off" a patient as being terminal.

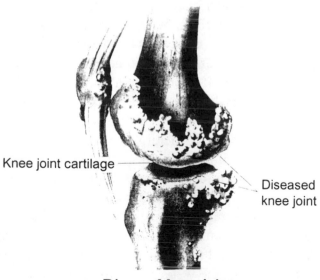

Knee joint cartilage

Diseased knee joint

**Diseased knee joint**

All of this I pointed out to Joe as we studied the joint diagram. "Look at these cartilage contact points," I said. "For one reason or another your cartilage has been wearing away. It takes time to cause the kind of damage your X-rays indicate. Apparently the process has been going on in your body for a long, long time . . ."

He nodded in agreement, looking somewhat frazzled. "Yeah, I know. That's what the surgeon told me. But, she didn't tell me why. Do *you* know why?"

"Joe, nobody can give you all the answers. And though, at this juncture, I can't tell you the exact triggering mechanism behind the problem, I can tell you this: Your cartilage contact points — right here — have been deprived for a long time of their crucial supply of synovial fluid, that your body makes from water. And that's resulted in a gradual, but steady rate of friction damage to your joints."

"And that's what wore my bone cartilage away?"

"That's the end result. But, there have been other reasons."

One of the difficulties faced by many health professionals is their tendency to treat individual symptoms as entities in and of themselves. When, in reality, the body is a unit, not a bunch of disparate parts. Therefore, any pain or malfunction, or any illness, is not, in and of itself, simply an isolated phenomenon. It is merely a local indicator of a systemic or general malfunction or deficiency of some kind.

For example, treating a headache with an aspirin, does not cure the cause. It merely treats the symptom. The aspirin doesn't know if it's being taken to relieve a headache, the pain of an ingrown toenail, or what. It simply affects — or treats — the central nervous system, which is involved in some degree with all major or minor disease conditions.

There's little doubt than any substance taken into the body affects the entire body. This is as true for the oxygen we breathe as it is for the water we drink. It is the body that makes the decision concerning how to handle — or dispose of — each and every substance we ingest.

Therefore, it is the body's intelligence, generally acknowledged to be the central nervous system (CNS), that determines what, and how much or little, of any substance the body can use, and where it is to be directed, utilized or stored. In other words, a single substance or nutrient (or drug) can have an incredible effect (or multiple effects) — positive or negative — upon the entire organism.

Using the same reasoning, the deficiency of a single substance or nutrient can produce enormous negative results to the entire body. And, depending upon a number of factors, including the age, sex, lifestyle, general health, environment, or the genetic makeup of an individual, that deficiency could produce either mild or devastating health or disease conditions.

As I shared this information with Joe, I quickly noted his eyes glaze over, either from disinterest or lack of understanding.

When I paused, he asked, "What does that have to do with arthritis?"

"That's a good question. The answer is: everything."

Joe had already told me about his early years: hard farm work in all kinds of weather conditions; college sports and resultant sports injuries. He'd also told me that he and his wife's busy lifestyle involved eating out most of the time, including frequent fast-food meals consisting of the Standard American Diet: burger, fries and soft drinks.

"And very few salads?"

"True. Very few of them. I've never liked rabbit food."

"Did you take food supplements, Joe? Vitamins, minerals and so on?"

He shook his head. "Nope. Didn't think I needed them. I've read that if you eat a balanced, nutritious diet that you don't need them . . ."

*Balanced . . . nutritious.*

"You are young, Joe, and for a good part of your life it seems that you've been relatively healthy . . . but, apparently something's been missing in your diet. And that's why you're body is breaking down."

"Breaking down?" he sounded alarmed.

"Breaking down. Wearing out. What you are experiencing are the typical symptoms of aging . . ."

I held up a second picture of an articular joint, similar to the one I had shown him earlier, the difference being that sketch picture clearly demonstrated both a dehydrated (dried

## *A well-hydrated and dehydrated joint - comparison*

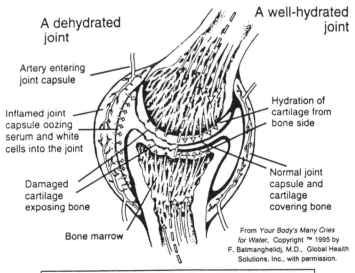

A dehydrated joint

A well-hydrated joint

Artery entering joint capsule

Hydration of cartilage from bone side

Inflamed joint capsule oozing serum and white cells into the joint

Damaged cartilage exposing bone

Normal joint capsule and cartilage covering bone

Bone marrow

From *Your Body's Many Cries for Water*, Copyright ™ 1995 by F. Batmanghelidj, M.D., Global Health Solutions, Inc., with permission.

Joint movement causes vacuum to be created within the joint space. Water will be pulled through the bone and the cartilage into the joint cavity - if it is freely available.

out) joint and a *well-hydrated* joint, side by side. "The left side is how your joint looks," I said. "Rough, exposed, damaged cartilage . . ."

Joe shuddered. "Yeah, bone grating against bone. That's my pain problem."

"You're exactly right. Now look at this right side of the picture."

The right of the picture portrayed a nutritionally healthy joint, with smooth, well-hydrated cartilage. "This is what your joints should look like."

The left side of the picture portrayed an inflamed, damaged cartilage. "This is the reason you have pain," I told Joe. "Because the cartilage is so rough. Instead of being well-padded, rounded and smooth — like the sketch on the right — your cartilage looks like a Montana road might look like in the spring time: all chewed up, with big chunks broken out of it."

*Cartilage health,* I told Joe, *is crucial to joint health.* Cartilage is the magical substance — smoother even than Teflon, five to eight times more slippery than ice — that's the key to the smooth, pain-free movement of our joints. As is most of the body, cartilage is a watery substance, 65% to 80% water. Water, in fact is vital to the efficient functioning of every cell and tissue of our bodies

Joe seriously studied both sides of the sketch, his face rather grim. Slowly he asked, "Is there *anything* that can be done about this?" Almost as quickly he brightened, and answered his own question, "That must mean I've got to drink more water . . ." He looked quite pleased with himself.

"Very good, Joe, you're catching on. The answer to your question is, Yes, something *can be done.* That's the *good* news. But, that's only part of the answer." Joe gestured impatiently. "It looks like you're just leading me on. *Can't you just give me something to make it better?*"

This is the total fallacy of the general view of health:

39

*instant healing*. All of the ads in magazines and on television promote the erroneous idea that for every pain and discomfort, there's a simple solution in a bottle, pill or capsule. And that every pain, discomfort, disease is simply a drug deficiency. But, it's not true.

*Turning any disease condition around is not that easy.*

"Not so fast, Joe. It's not easy. It's true that your arthritic condition *can be reversed*. And I can help you . . . I can guide you in doing it. But, how well it can be done, and how quickly your body will respond . . . well, that's totally another story. And it's mostly up to you."

He squirmed nervously. "Okay. Okay, Dr. Bob. I'm not trying to jump the gun. But, I've suffered too much, for too long. And I'm anxious to get on with it. Tell me what I've got to do. Give it to me straight. I'm ready . . . I'm ready to go."

In a nutshell, I told him, correcting, reversing, healing arthritis *is as simple and as difficult as* correcting the entire body's metabolic balance.

Why is this so? As referred to earlier, a person suffering from any complaint or health challenge, or disease, tends to focus on the symptoms he or she feels or sees. What is almost always overlooked is the fact that a person having arthritic symptoms is usually (practically always) suffering from general deterioration of health. This can be in the form of (most prevalent) overwhelming fatigue; sluggish or poor digestion; poor elimination, such as chronic constipation, and so on.

The basic solution to arthritis (or any disease condition) is to totally turn around and correct the metabolic imbalance(s). This involves a corrective program.

Joe insisted he was "ready for anything" that could or would ease or correct his symptoms and help produce relief from pain. ". . . and make me healthy again!"

"First," I told him, "I'm going to introduce you to the interesting world of essential fatty acids . . . and fatty degeneration."

He raised his eyebrows. "Essential *fatty* acids? Fatty *degeneration?* You were just giving me a bad time about the fat in my burger and fries . . ."

"That's true," I admitted, "I was. But not all fats and oils are harmful. Some are an absolute necessity. Without a certain amount of fats and oils in our diets, we would become ill and die . . ."

"Sounds like a paradox to me," Joe quipped.

"Not really. In general terms, it's either the hard fats, the fats that don't melt at room temperatures, or the fats and oils that have been altered in processing, that are the bad fats. And . . . or," I went on, "by the good fats and oils that have become bad or rancid. This condition is known as fatty degeneration. The great killer diseases of our time, the ones we frequently call 'degenerative diseases,' such as cardiovascular disease, cancer, diabetes, obesity, multiple sclerosis (MS), fatty deposits in the inner organs, such as liver and kidneys, some emotional and behavioral problems — *and arthritis* — all involve fatty degeneration."

"Clarify for me, what, exactly is fatty degeneration?"

"That's a condition involving a lack or imbalance of essential fatty acids and/or the presence of altered (hydrogenated) fatty materials in places (such as inside the cells) or quantities in which they are not normally found," I told him.

"And this condition is serious? "Joe asked.

"I'll let you answer your own question: Is arthritis serious? Heart disease? Or cancer, and so on? As I said, Joe, all of these degenerative conditions are in some way connected with, or lack of, essential fatty acids."

41

## Chapter Five
## THE FATTY ACIDS

My research has led me to believe that *the study of fatty acids could well be the key to unlock the secrets of health.* Fatty acids deal with health at the cellular level. They are basic, key ingredients to life itself. Without fatty acids, cells as living, functioning units could not, would not exist. Fatty acids are the main components of the membranes that surround every cell in our bodies.

Fatty acids play starring roles in the construction and maintenance of all healthy cells and the membranes within the cells, including even the subminiature subcellular organelles themselves. I pulled out my cell diagram and studied it.

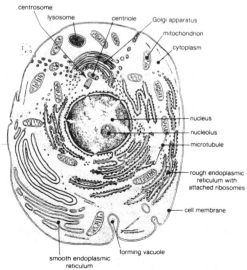

**Typical human cell**

Life at the cellular level — which is actually where it's lived — is awesome. Truly, our life is in our cells. Microscopic in size, they are billions of times more dynamic, powerful and explosive than any atomic explosion. Each single cell is an entity unto itself, a powerhouse of activity and productivity; a unique creation that would stagger even the wildest Jules Verne flight of imagination. An incredible combination of autonomy and democracy, the intelligence and wisdom of these subminiature energy factories is beyond the capability of our minds to comprehend or to describe.

I traced the boundaries of the diagram with my finger. "This is where your life is lived, Joe," I said. "Not in your head. Not in your brain. But, here. In each one of these miraculous little creations."

He nodded. "Yeah, but . . .?"

"You want to know what all this's got to do with you and your arthritis?"

"Exactly. I don't get the connection."

I chuckled. "That's what I thought your reaction would be."

Thinking that a lecture was on its way, Joe shifted uncomfortably in his chair. He was right. I knew I could not effectively help him institute a healing nutritional regime until he understood the basics. I tried another tack.

"Tell me, Joe, what did you have for lunch?"

"Lunch? What are you getting at?" Joe asked, slightly irritated.

"You did eat?" I pushed.

"Yeah, sure. Well, I was in a hurry, so I stopped at the . . ." A flush of red showed above his collar and spread across his face.

"Go on. What did you eat? Something . . . in a hurry?"

He sighed. "You got me. It was a cheeseburger, a shake and fries."

"Okay, Joe, let me tell you something. I don't have a microscope here, but if I did, I could predict what you would see in a drop of your blood. Would you like to know? Really?"

"Well, yes, I guess I would. What would you see?"

"First of all, within minutes the fat you'd just eaten would show up in your blood. But, that's only part of it."

I stabbed a finger at the cell picture before us. "Right here, Joe, interfering with the cell membrane's permeability . . . would be tiny little droplets of fat. And some of those droplets of fat would get through into the cell . . ." I looked directly into his eyes. "Then, Joe, do you know what would happen — is happening right now?"

Again he shifted uncomfortably in his seat. "No. What?"

"When the individual cells of your cellular system, get clogged with the saturated fat from the beef in your hamburger and the oil in your fries, well . . ."

"Well, what?"

"Then they'll get sick. And if the problem isn't turned around, they'll die."

"They'll die?"

I had his attention now. "That's right, Joe. When the cellular membranes get clogged with hard fats or oils, such as those in your burger and fries, they lose some, or all of their ability to become permeated with oxygen . . . and that's serious."

I paused for emphasis. "And, Joe, you know that you can't live for very long without oxygen. That *you*, is *all of you, including each individual cell.*"

I leaned back in my chair, waiting for him to respond.

"But, Dr. Bob, I've had meals like that hundreds of times . . . and it never seemed to bother me . . ." He stopped short, a look of comprehension upon his face. "At least I didn't think then that it did . . ."

45

Apparently he was doing more serious thinking than he'd done in a long, long time. Suddenly his face brightened. "Are you trying to tell me something?"

I nodded, but didn't speak.

"What is it? Are you trying to tell me that my eating habits are responsible for my health?"

I laughed and slapped him on the shoulder. "Absolutely!"

"But, some of the doctors I went to told me that food had nothing to do with my health . . . or my arthritis."

"Well, it does, Joe. In fact, what did you think your body was built on?"

"I guess I never really thought much about it."

"Joe, your body is built of food . . . and water . . . and air . . . and sunlight. That's all. Nothing more and nothing less."

That was the turn-around day for Joe James. Up until that time he'd been more interested in *philosophically discussing* his situation; getting acquainted, and learning to trust me. But that day he seemed to begin accepting his role in taking responsibility for himself and his well-being. I believed that he was ready. So I seriously began educating him: concerning the vital importance of his diet — about fats and oils, essential fatty acids and prostaglandins — and the health- and life-sustaining functions that these unique nutrients perform in our bodies.

That was also the day that Joe asked for and I gave him an outline of the basic items that his health — and his very life — depended upon.

"To begin with," I began, "there are several families of fatty acids . . . and they come in many shapes and sizes."

Fatty acids are so tiny that 100 quintillion of them (or 100 followed by 18 zeroes) are present in a single drop of oil, yet they exert enormous influence in every function of every cell, tissue and organ of the body. There are two basic kinds of fatty acids: saturated and unsaturated.

*Saturated fatty acids* are the simplest fatty acids and are found in all food fats and oils. They are especially abundant in hard fats, or fats that are solid at room temperatures. Although the body needs a certain amount of saturated fatty acids, to generate energy, construct membranes or to make unsaturated fatty acids, an excess can cause health problems for our hearts and arteries. Our bodies can also store saturated fatty acids in our tissues for future use.

*Unsaturated fatty acids* are liquid oils. While saturated fatty acids tend to aggregate and stick together . . .

I grinned at Joe. "*Saturated* fatty acids . . . they were the fats you ingested in the burger and fries you ate today."

He grimaced, but said nothing.

"This, of course," I went on, "causes problems for our arteries and hearts. And since unsaturated fatty acids tend to disperse, to move apart, to be anti-sticky, they are the fats that perform important chemical and transport functions . . ."

"Transport functions?" Joe broke in. "What are they?"

"Transport means to carry . . . unsaturated fatty acids are so fluid they can move into and out of our cells, helping to carrying nutrients into the cells and waste matter out. There's no way to emphasize the crucial importance of these functions: one to nutrify, the other to detoxify our bodies. The hindering of either would put our health at risk . . ."

Although there are many fatty acids in the body, saturated and unsaturated, only two of them carry the special distinction of being *essential*. These are Omega 3 and Omega 6. Essential means our bodies must have them, cannot make them, therefore must obtain them from food. They must come from the foods and other nutrients we ingest.

Significantly, it is estimated that 60% to 95% of the population is deficient in one or more essential fatty acids (EFAs); making it no surprise, that the resulting disease conditions are called *diseases of fatty acid degeneration.*

"You've got to have a daily supply of both," I told Joe, "Omega 3 and Omega 6 . . . do you understand why?"

"I think so, but remind me."

"Because, they're so chemically active . . . that's why. They attract oxygen, sort of like a magnet attracts iron filings, and pull it into our bodies. And the need for oxygen is, of course, obvious. There are many reasons why EFAs are so vital to our health. But they can all be spelled out in six small words: *They are the fats that heal . . .*"

I paused for emphasis. And for a moment we were both silent. Then Joe came up with the question which should have been obvious by now.

"Are you telling me that fatty acids heal *everything*? I've got arthritis, not heart disease or artery disease. Do fatty acids also heal arthritis?"

"The answer is yes. Directly and indirectly. Because, along with everything else they do, essential fatty acids produce prostaglandins."

Joe sighed deeply and made a face. "Prosta . . . prosta? I can't even pronounce the word. What in the world are prostaglandins?"

I laughed. "It's not hard to pronounce. Just think of prostate. The prostate gland. That's what they are named after."

Prostaglandins, named for the gland from which they were first isolated, in the prostate gland of sheep, are short-lived chemicals that regulate cellular activities on a moment-to-moment basis. Prostaglandins are *extremely powerful entities that affect every aspect of every person's health* (male and female alike). Our bodies make prostaglandins, PGs for short, from essential fatty acids or EFAs.

There are over 30 different PGs that have presently been isolated and identified. But, in context, it's the prostaglandin nicknamed PG1, that we're most interested in at the moment.

Although PG1s work an impressive list of miracles in our bodies, such as — keeping blood platelets from sticking together — a condition known as "sludging" — (which helps prevent heart attacks and strokes) . . .

**Sludging after a fatty meal reduces oxygen in the blood.**

Prostaglandin PG2 is largely responsible for a condition known as "sludging" in which circulating fats in the blood cause red cells to become sticky. Cells must remain flexible and move freely to carry oxygen and nutrients to the tiny capillaries (as in A). Within one hour following a fatty meal (B) cell movement has slowed. Within six hours sludging has become so severe that blood flow stops in small blood vessels. Eight hours after a fatty meal (C) cell stickiness is evident in even the larger vessels. Sludging can lead to strokes and serious heart conditions.

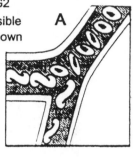
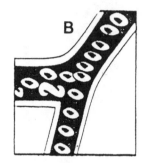
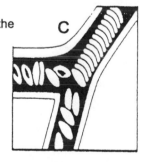

. . . by helping remove sodium and excess fluids from our body; relaxing blood vessels to improve circulation; helping diabetics by making insulin work better; and improving nerve function, which helps to relieve anxiety and depression and gives us a sense of well-being.

Plus a few other various and assorted miraculous functions.

Nothing on this list had Joe exactly jumping up and down.

Not until I gave him the bottom line.

"You're going to love this one, Joe. PG1s decrease the body's inflammation response. And that's how *PG1s help control arthritis.*"

## Chapter Six
## THE CURE

According to numerous biological health professionals, cardiovascular disease and some types of diabetes are not difficult to cure. And *arthritis* — one of the most prevalent disease conditions in the Western world — along with allergies, asthma, migraines and many other conditions respond well to nutrient enrichment, improved digestion, selection of compatible foods, and detoxification.

One of the first, and certainly the most prominent health professional to deal with arthritis on a nutritional basis was Paavo Airola, who went public in his book, *There Is a Cure for Arthritis*, which was published in 1968. Based on the sales of Dr. Airola's book, a rather large number of people read and heeded his nutritional guidance; but, for so-called mainstream medicine, his protocol was ignored.

Utilizing Dr. Airola's insights and others, I have helped guide several arthritis sufferers into paths of understanding the causes of their suffering, and pointed them in the direction of healing themselves. Some have heeded. For most, though, accepting responsibility for their own health proved too much to handle.

I hoped Joe would not be one of the latter. Though he did begin bravely, as many others have done, he did appear to be making good progress. For how long, it was anybody's guess. Perhaps fortuitously, it was at this juncture that my path crossed with that of Dr. David Allen.

With an educational background almost as diverse as the universe itself Dr. Allen is a personal wellness consultant

51

to celebrities, business leaders and world-renowned athletes. Along with his wife Barbara, who is a Women's Health Advocate and educator, David Allen is co-founder of Quantum Connection, Inc., a corporation that specializes in product formulations, unique raw materials, proprietary products and marketing strategies for the Natural Health Care Industry.

The three of us met during the process of producing a life-extension audio-tape, and formed an instant affinity for each other. Some time after we had finished production of the tape, I received a telephone call from David. I listened with growing excitement as he informed me that his company had just produced and was in the beginning stages of marketing a "revolutionary, proprietary new product that is extremely effective against all forms of arthritis: CM Pure™."

And, would I be interested in sharing the product with some of my friends or family who might be suffering from arthritis? Would I?

"Absolutely. I have somebody in mind right this minute."

David chuckled at my response. "Most people do. So I'll ship you a bottle of CM Pure™ for you to evaluate any way you'd like."

Just prior to this conversation with David Allen, Joe had embarked upon a specially-designed nutritional program in an attempt to begin controlling his arthritis, which was steadily getting worse.

When David's package arrived, I quickly examined the attractively-labeled bottle of CM Pure™, and immediately passed it on to my friend. I eagerly awaited for the response. I didn't have to wait long. A little over two weeks later, I received the more than enthusiastic report: "Not only did CM Pure™ relieve my pain, but I can now walk up stairs without assistance. That's something I haven't done in ages."

When I relayed this information to David Allen he was delighted. "That's the same kind of reports we've been getting every day!"

*However, David Allen informed me, it had taken them many months of agonizing effort for them to attain these kind of results.*

It was early in 1995 when Dr. David and Barbara Allen first learned of the long-chain fatty acid cetyl ester that was to so dramatically impact their lives. Dr. David Allen is a nutritionist-researcher who specializes in -- among many other things -- the research and development of antioxidants and essential fatty acids.

Knowing Dr. Allen's interest in fatty acids, one of the manufacturers with whom he was working at the time passed on a bit of information about "a new fatty acid." Allen was intrigued and did some checking. What he learned convinced him that *this had to be one of the most unique long-chain fatty acids yet discovered.* He began working to see if he could produce sufficient quantities to test it.

Allen certainly knew what he was talking about. Well-versed in biological medicine, he had done extensive research on Evening Primrose Oil, along with a considerable amount of time studying fatty acids in general, as well as the essential fatty acids, Omega 3 and Omega 6.

"So, when this unique long-chain fatty acid came to my attention," David said, "I was already conversant with the fatty acid mechanisms, their relationship to prostaglandins, and how they affect every cell in the human body."

As a scientist, Allen was fully aware of the problems related to the diets that are high in saturated fats and trans-fatty acids that are common to most Americans.

"I believe," he said, "that such diets could and very likely do become triggering mechanisms for arthritis and other diseases of fatty degeneration, such as cardiovascular disease, diabetes, multiple sclerosis, kidney degeneration, liver degeneration and others, all of which have increased dramatically in the past 100 years . . ."

*Arthritis — the Crippler — is one of America's most dreaded diseases, and is caused, at least in part, by fatty degeneration at the cellular level!*

The Food and Drug Administration (FDA) has apparently never approved a drug that will cure arthritis, and the drugs they have approved have multiple side effects. If the FDA had approved a drug that would cure arthritis, some 50 million Americans would not be suffering from arthritis today.

Arthritis causes more suffering and disfigurement than any other disease condition. It can disfigure hands, twist spines, paralyze joints, weaken connective tissue in the heart and other vital organs; the most damaging being to the kidneys and liver. Arthritis can also cause fatigue, intense depression and agonizing pain.

In 1982 the FDA withdrew a drug from the market that had caused 12 deaths; and from that date till the present has removed still other so-called arthritis drugs which have caused severe side effects and more deaths. A few of these FDA approved drugs may help ease the pain of arthritis, but taken over a long period of time will compound the existing arthritic damage with their harmful side effects.

The cost to each user can run into thousands of dollars, merely palliating the disease, but not curing it. For the most part doctors' treatments are only as effective as the products researchers give them to work with.

By May of 1996 Allen cautiously began sharing the new fatty acid with a few people who were suffering from rheumatoid arthritis and osteoarthritis, and a few related conditions that seemed to be indicated.

To his chagrin, the results he hoped and expected were not forthcoming. Some people felt better. Others felt worse. It was extremely frustrating.

Yet, based on his knowledge of biochemistry, David Allen believed that in principle this fatty acid cetyl ester should work. But it wasn't until some time later that he learned why the product had not performed according to his expectations, and exactly how to configure a unique, long-chain fatty acid cetyl ester so as to exceed even his fondest dreams for it.

CM Pure™, derived from the tropical rain forest, is an evolutionary advancement over earlier generations of long-chain fatty acid cetyl ester products. This is basically because CM Pure™ is a biologically-effective plant-based product that is transformed and concentrated when made into a powder by Quantum Botanicals.

CM Pure™ was photographed using Chris Wedtke's modern Kirlian photography method. The results were truly astounding. CM Pure™ exhibited a very strong essential energy and life force that's inherent in its product.

When superfoods like CM Pure™ are balanced, the electromagnetic vibrational energies become a part of the person who ingests them, significantly increasing the efficacy and healing potential of the product.

## Chapter Seven
## THE CM PURE™ STORY

What happened then was to be for Dr. David and Barbara Allen  the realization of the American Dream. They had found a need; they were convinced that they had found a way (and a product) to meet that need. *All they had to do now was to perfect that product.*

How were they to do that?

After serious soul searching and considerable thought, David called a close friend of his, Dr. B. P. Poovaiah. The inclusion of Poovaiah in the project was a stroke of genius. With his extensive training — two Master's degrees, one in Horticulture and Botany, another in Food Technology, plus a Ph.D. in Nutritional Biochemistry — along with many years of experience in dietary supplement industries, Dr. Poovaiah proved to be just the man to help them come up with viable answers to the very hard questions they were asking themselves.

First: Why didn't the long-chain fatty acid cetyl ester formulation they tried to market meet their expectations? Was something wrong with the formulation?

Second: How could they take this "diamond-in-the -rough" compound and make it so good that it would exceed even their expectations?

Third: How could they perfect an anti-inflammatory/ auto-immune product that would end arthritic suffering for millions?

Fourth: Could it be done, and could they do it?

57

*Hard questions that demanded clear-cut, definitive answers.* That they did do it is testified to by the thousands who have already tried and benefited from the results of their labors. *How they accomplished all this is a story unto itself.*

Early research had proved that the purer the fatty acid ester used, the more dramatic the results would be. That, David Allen realized, must be one of the keys to the solution of their problem. Allen learned that the product they had been using was derived from beef tallow and contained only a very small amount of the active ingredient. It is Dr. Allen's policy not to criticize or "knock" competitive products, because in the final analysis, the true test of any product's worth is based on its effectiveness with the end consumer.

Convinced that a pure source of a long-chain fatty acid cetyl ester would achieve the healing results they desired, they determined to locate a natural plant source. It took months of extensive research and expensive investment in technological equipment to do so, but they finally achieved their declared goal: The unparalleled, highly effective CM Pure™.

Dr. Allen had CM Pure™ analyzed by Covance Laboratories of Madison, Wisconsin (a national certified testing laboratory). CM Pure™ was administered to a group of test animals to evaluate its toxicity in accordance with the Federal Drug Administration Good Laboratory Practice Regulations, 21 CFR 58. All procedures used were in compliance with the Animal Welfare Act Regulations. All animals appeared normal throughout the study period and no mortalities occurred. CM Pure™ is definitely a safe product.

Dr. B. P. Poovaiah is probably one of the world's foremost authorities on fatty acids, especially essential fatty acids. Early in his career Poovaiah conducted some of the original research on Omega 3. While serving as a doctoral and faculty member at the University of California in Berkeley and San Francisco Medical School during the 60s

58

and 70s Poovaiah led a research team of scientists that proved the importance of Omega 3.

Prior to that time Omega 3 was considered to be just another fatty acid without any particular nutritional implications. Dr. Poovaiah and his colleague proved that Omega 3 is an *essential* fatty acid, ranking in importance with Omega 6.

In addition to his work with Omega 3, Poovaiah has also done extensive research on Omega 6 and Omega 9. Because of his extensive work with fatty acids, Poovaiah knew a great deal about both the acute and chronic forms of inflammatory and immune response causes.

*He was also well versed in his knowledge of the arthritic disease process.*

"Then Poovaiah was just the right man for you . . . at precisely the right time," I remarked to David Allen. "And with him on board, you were able to operate much more effectively. Right?"

"Exactly," David said. "With joining us, to focus his considerable technical and research ability on producing a pure product, I believed it would be only a matter of time before we would have the breakthrough we needed."

Once again, David's instincts were right.

"So you did it," I said. "You and your team achieved that long-sought breakthrough?"

"Yes . . . yes, we did."

"Then what happened?"

David's face glowed as he told me, "This discovery has enabled us to take a quantum leap beyond all of the other products in the marketplace . . .!"

*The essence of that breakthrough — the research and development of a plant-based, long-chain fatty acid cetyl ester product — might very well determine the manner in which all arthritis and other inflammatory and auto-immune*

59

*diseases will be treated well into the next century, and even beyond!*

With an estimated 50,000,000 Americans victims of osteoarthritis; 6,000,000 afflicted with rheumatoid arthritis (no one can even guess the number of world-wide sufferers of arthritis in its many forms) — and the actual cause(s) of the disease a mystery — it's evident the world is definitely ready for a breakthrough of any kind.

In my research and lecture travels across the United States and abroad, I have become increasingly aware of the world's burgeoning urgent health needs. Every where I go I am besieged with urgent request for help, for information: "My pain is unbearable . . . what can I do about it?" "Please help me."

For a number of years I was a journalist and editor on the staff of World Vision International, and as such I beheld sights that I had only heard of before: the blind, the lame and the crippled. At that time I could do little to ease the vast amount of suffering I encountered.

Since then I have become trained to recognize that much of the sickness and pain we are surrounded with come as a result of ignorance. Ignorance of the nutritional needs of our bodies. When the basic nutritional needs are not known or understood, or ignored, pain and sickness results.

The same is true of arthritis. Medical doctors and scientists realize that synthetic drugs do not heal arthritis and that they serve only to treat and to ease the pain.

What was needed, I realized, was a natural product, one made from plant sources. One that not only eased the pain, but furnished the body with substances that help rebuild damaged tissues. CM Pure™ is just such a product.

Having suffered for many years with spinal problems, when CM Pure™ first became available, I was eager to try it. When I did, I quickly joined the ranks of lthose who had personally experienced the product's "incredible results."

The "incredible results" I personally experienced are the same type of results David Allen and Poovaiah were so pleased with.

There was much that I didn't know about the diseases of arthritis and what could constitute a cure, so I met and interviewed Dr. B. P. Poovaiah.

"Why," I asked him, "are you so interested in the science of nutrition?"

"Because, we believe that arthritis is in some way connected to or affected by good nutrition," he told me.

"Has science actually blamed arthritis upon some dietary deficiency?"

He shook his head. "Not precisely. Although no dietary deficiency has been proven to be causally related to RA, it seems to be clear that the disease is a chronic progressive inflammatory tissue disorder in which good nutrition of an individual is of fundamental importance."

"Additionally," Poovaiah said, "a recent review of rheumatoid arthritis points out that symptoms of the disease begin only when three conditions develop: First, macrophages and activated T lymphocytes release cytokines; followed by the development of a network of blood vessels in the synovial membrane; and the invasion of neutrophils into the joint cavity."

"And you, along with Dr. Allen and Dr. Johnson believe that fatty acids with an appropriate combination of catalysts could in some way be involved in the alleviating or preventing of this scenario, the arthritis inflammatory process?" I asked him.

Poovaiah nodded. "We are certain of it."

"Do you have some historical data regarding this?"

"Actually, yes. In fact as early as the year 1800, fish oil, which is a fatty acid, was being used in London, England. They found it to be very useful in the treatment and curing of rickets and arthritis at the Manchester Infirmary in London."

Even though this information was reported in the *London Medical Journal* of 1783, it has taken centuries for such facts to surface and to be  scientifically fully understood.

"Was that fact what sparked your interest in fatty acids as they relate to arthritis?"

Poovaiah smiled. "Well, I've been interested in fatty acids for a long time. I have always felt there's much more to them than what is generally known. When that bit of information came to my attention, it simply whetted my interest in fatty acids . . . especially as they relate to arthritis and other inflammatory conditions."

"So you decided to delve into the matter."

"That's about right."

"But," I countered, "hasn't there been a great deal known about fatty acids for a long time?"

"Yes, but not enough."

"It seems to me that other scientists would have focused on fatty acids," I said. "Is there any particular reason why they didn't?"

"Yes, there's a very good reason.  To do research work with fats and oils such as I did, you have to work with powerful acids and toxic solvents. It's potentially very dangerous. It's hard work. Meticulous work . . ."

"Then you have to use protective devices . . .?"

"Yes, mask and other protective garb. All of that.

"But the work has been rewarding," Dr. Poovaiah went on. "Among other facts my research has turned up, is that in arthritic patients it is now known that leukotrienes and cytokines are affected by consumption of fish oil . . ."

"Leukotrienes?  And  cytokines?"  I  interrupted. "Exactly what are they?"

Dr. Poovaiah patiently explained, "It gets a trifle complex. But, basically, leukotrienes are a class of peptolipids derived from arachidonic acid. And cytokines are small proteins or polypeptides produced by immunocytes. For example: T-cells, monocytes/macrophages and fibroblasts. They function in hormone-like fashion in cell-to-cell communication . . .

"Although cytokines are important entities for our immune systems, they are a mixed blessing. Even though cytokines do mediate or assist our immune responses, they may also be responsible for harmful tissue destruction, enhanced inflammation and proliferation of cells in blood vessel walls."

"Why is this information important to arthritis research?" I asked.

"Because cytokines are present in the joint fluids of arthritic patients. Not just one kind, but several of them."

"And that's bad?"

"It's not good."

"What do you mean by that?"

By the way Poovaiah patiently tried to simplify for me some complicated biochemistry principles, I can believe he would be an excellent professor. "Exactly how cytokines contribute to rheumatoid arthritis is not known," he said.

"However, it appears that some of them orchestrate the metabolic responses that follow immune system provocation, or injury. Laboratory studies of interleukin-1 cytokines prove that they increase collagenase synthesis, stimulate T-cell activity, and are believed to activate leukocytes and stimulate fibrosis . . . *all of which contribute to the inflammatory and degradatory processes observed in rheumatoid arthritis.*"

I was wondering how fatty acids would come into the picture. It seemed, I reasoned, that any action that could reduce interleukin-1 production and modulate cytokine responses could be expected to diminish the symptoms of rheumatoid arthritis and retard its progress.

Poovaiah's next words confirmed my assumptions. "Studies have shown," he said, "with both healthy and arthritic subjects that *consumption of fish oil reduces the production of interleukin-1 and modulates cytokine responses*. In other words, fish oils offer some improvement in rheumatoid arthritis. More importantly, they do this without serious side effects."

Again, I wondered why. And again, Dr. Poovaiah answered my question with his next words. "That's because fish oil contains EFA long-chain fatty acids."

"Then, fish oil should be the answer to arthritis. Right?"

He smiled again. "You might think so. But that's not always the case. You see, in spite of all of the positive benefits of fish oil in the arthritic situation, not all arthritic patients respond to fish oil treatment. Which means, that for many arthritic persons their inability to benefit from fish oil has left them with no other recourse than to resort to the use of drugs."

I sat musing for a moment on how that culturally, we have become trained to expect instant healing from all pain and inflammation, much as we are trained to expect instant gratification of all our needs and desires. However, our bodies don't work that way. When provided with the necessary raw materials, our bodies effectively attain, regain and maintain our body's health through layers of specific cell groups — a process that takes time.

Drugs work quickly, often dramatically, but generally produce problems of their own, such as the "rebound effect," or reoccurrence of the symptoms when the drugs are withdrawn.

"And," I said somewhat ruefully, "even at their best, and when used in the most advantageous manner, drugs are generally immune suppressing agents.

"Unlike CM Pure™," I continued my musing aloud, "and other essential fatty acids, that strive to attain and maintain the body's homeostasis or equilibrium, drugs do interfere with homeostasis by antagonizing the crucial participation of prostaglandins, and thus prevent the completion of their biochemical reaction . . .

"How wonderful that today, with the development and availability of CM Pure™, the use of NSAIDs and other anti-inflammatory drugs are no longer   necessarily the arthritis treatment of choice."

Now I came to the question I'd been waiting to ask. "Dr. Poovaiah, in your precise scientific opinion, what is CM Pure™? What is its essence and the mechanism by which it works? In other words, how does CM Pure™  fit into the arthritis picture?"

In his brief and to the point answer, Dr. Poovaiah told me that CM Pure™ consists of long-chain fatty acids similar, though not identical, to the fatty acids found in fish oil . . .

"CM Pure™," he said, "is formulated by a special proprietary process, the inter-esterification of a long chain fatty acid with cetyl alcohol in the presence of some important catalysts. This produces a biologically active compound that's both safe and effective as a dietary supplement.

"In many ways CM Pure™ perhaps has the ability to interfere with interleuken production and modulate cytokine response . . ."

My accumulated research was coming together in my mind. "Does that mean that CM Pure™ is an anti-inflammatory compound?"

"Perhaps," Poovaiah responded. "CM Pure™ — by some as yet unknown mechanism — helps to mediate and balance cellular and tissue inflammation, heat, redness, swelling and pain. It may be doing this biochemically

65

through the help of *prostaglandins*, those short-lived hormone-like chemicals I mentioned a few minutes ago.

"The good prostaglandins that regulate the powerful immune response functions of the immune system. And, as you know, without the benefits of an efficiently-functioning immune system, our bodies would be defenseless against various entities that would make us ill . . ."

"What about the other prostaglandins, the bad ones?"

"Oh, yes, the bad ones. With respect to the condition of arthritis, they're the ones that come from arachidonic acid. Well, CM Pure™ very effectively inhibits the inflammatory pathways caused by arachadonic acid. And this makes CM Pure™ *the most potent fatty acid yet discovered, and the catalyst for blocking the metabolic pathways responsible for inflammation.*"

CM Pure™, I was learning, has the ability to interfere with inflammatory reactions, which are necessary if muscles are to undergo repeated contraction. CM Pure™ removes muscle weakness by promoting protein synthesis around joints. Further, long-chain fatty acids — CM Pure™ and others — are and become constituents of cell membranes and are stored in membrane phospholipids, making them readily available as precursors of several metabolic pathways for future use.

"All of this is critically important, but CM Pure™ not only contains long-chain fatty acids, but other catalysts as well, making it powerful enough to handle those challenges. In rheumatoid arthritis conditions, for example, CM Pure™ can induce many biochemical changes in ground substances and even alter the responses of connective tissues, similar to those produced by some steroid drug treatment . . ."

My antenna went up. "Steroid drugs? What about side effects?"

"Good catch," Poovaiah said. "There is a difference. CM Pure™ has no known side effects such as is the case with steroid drugs . . ."

I was still thinking. "Steroids? But doesn't our bodies produce steroids?"

"Absolutely. Our bodies do produce steroid hormones. They produce them from cholesterol . . ."

"From cholesterol?"

Poovaiah chuckled. "Of course. And without those natural steroid hormones, we wouldn't be able to tell a male from a female. Because the best known steroid hormones are the female hormones estrogen and progesterone, and the male hormone testosterone . . . and normally these cause no side effects."

"What about synthetic hormones, the steroids that athletes use?"

Those steroids, the anabolic steroids, such as those used by athletes, are dangerous. They are synthetically produced male steroid hormones, and are known to have serious side effects like liver, brain, kidney, ligament and joint damage. They can also cause cancer. Whereas, as mentioned above, CM Pure™, being a naturally-produced fatty acid compound, causes no side effects whatsoever.

"There are other entities that may work with CM Pure™ to keep our bodies healthy. For example, there are the eicosanoids . . ." Poovaiah began.

I interrupted him. "Eicosanoids? What are they and what do they do that could have a positive effect upon our health, especially someone with arthritis?"

As usual, Poovaiah was patient with me.

"Eicosanoids," he began, "are strong, short-lived hormone-like compounds that are derived from oxygenation of long-chain fatty acids, somewhat similar to CM Pure™. They lead a very fleeting existence, lasting for mere seconds, or at the most, minutes.

"But in that brief moment of time eicosanoids achieve powerful results, such as: dilating blood vessels and increassing blood flow, inducing powerful muscle contractions, and attracting leukocytes to sites of inflammation."

Later I was to learn that these will-o'-the-wisp eicosanoids truly exercise a great deal of power in our bodies. They can modulate hypothalamic and pituitary release of hormones, and may even have the ability to rapidly alter cell function themselves. They are capable of triggering release of collagen, regulating cell and tissue functions, secretory activity, smooth muscle behavior and cell-to-cell interactions.

*All of these are actions and functions that help relieve the pain and sufferings of arthritic conditions.*

"So you see," Poovaiah went on, "CM Pure™ helps indirectly to keep our bodies in a healthy condition in a number of different ways. It helps make it possible for our bodies to build and maintain better, more permeable cell membranes, both the semi-permeable external cell membrane, as well as all of the cell's internal entities or organelles. CM Pure™ is involved in all of this. A truly wonderful product.

"To sum it up," Poovaiah said, "testimonials from those using CM Pure™ indicate that it provides outstanding benefits to every person (and *every body*), especially those suffering from arthritis and any other type of inflammatory tissue condition."

I came away from my time with Dr. Poovaiah with a greater understanding of CM Pure™. When I returned to my office, I made a brief outline of some of the compound's benefits, which include in part:

• CM Pure™ makes possible the efficient, selective transfer of vital nutrients through the cell membranes into the cell.

- CM Pure™ increases the permeability of internal cell structures which enables the cell to more efficiently extract nutrients from the blood stream and to dispose of cellular waste substances.
- CM Pure™ helps to create osmolarity of cellular fluids and helps to open the cellular channels.
- CM Pure™ benefits extend to and include every membrane of every cell in every tissue and organ.
- CM Pure™ benefits include all cells, including the bone cells of the cartilage, *thus directly assisting the body's ability to regenerate and heal arthritis-damaged cartilage and surrounding tissue.*
- CM Pure™ improves cell-to-cell communication.
- CM Pure™ closely resembles fish oil, but has far more powerful, long-lasting effects on the body.
- CM Pure™ helps normalize hyperimmune responses found in rheumatoid arthritis.
- CM Pure™ acts as a surfactant (surface acting agent) and a powerful anti-inflammatory agent.
- CM Pure™ can be very economical, especially for the seriously-afflicted, who may spend hundreds of dollars a month on medications for their arthritis.
- As a plant-based product, CM Pure™ produces no negative side effects.

## Chapter Eight
## AFRICA'S RAIN FOREST/CHINA CONNECTION

"Africa," says A. Kweku Andoh, "may yet come forth in all its pristine glory, to show the world that it could change the entire course of history . . ."

These are not idle words.

Dr. Andoh knows whereof he speaks. Born in the tropical rain forests of Ghana, Andoh is a British-educated ethnobotanist and a Fellow of the Linnean Society of London. He is among the world's foremost ethnobotanists. He works closely with Drs. Allen and Poovaiah on the CM Pure™ Project and speaks throughout the world on behalf of the world's endangered rain forests.

"At least 75 percent of our oxygen is derived from these forests," Dr. Andoh told me. "And at the rate we are destroying our rain forests, the world will soon find itself gasping for oxygen . . ."

It is common knowledge that hundreds of acres of these precious natural resources are being destroyed each day, and that the world's ecosystems are suffering from the thousands of tons of toxic wastes being poured into the oceans and atmosphere. But what is not as generally known, is that *many of the antidotes for the poisons created by the industrial world,* are stored in the deep recesses of the tropical rain forests.

Descendant of a long line of botanists, herbalists and traditional healers for many generations Dr. Anthony Kweku Andoh has committed his considerable talents and resources to make those wonderful rain forest remedies available

71

through David Allen to help bring healing to the world. Quantum Botanicals has allocated a percentage of the company's profits to the African Rain Forest Foundation for the purpose of protecting numerous species of healing plants by helping to fund a botanical garden in Ghana that will cultivate and preserve endangered plants.

Dr. David and Barbara Allen have also formed an alliance with Ethnobotanist Richard Fontes, who has spent over a decade in developing the rich resources of the Peruvian and Amazonian rain forests.

On yet another continent -- China -- David Allen is cooperating with his long-time friend, Dr. T. Colin Campbell, by helping promote Campbell's Biomar diagnostic technology for the prediction of cancer, cardiovascular and other degenerative diseases, which can be detected years prior to the appearance of any symptoms.

This ground-breaking technology has grown out of what has been termed the China-Cornell-Oxford Project on Nutrition, Environment and Health. First in 1983 and again in 1989, headed by Dr. Campbell, American, Chinese and English researchers gathered information on how people live and die in 65 counties in various parts of China.

*The result of these efforts has been the most comprehensive database on the multiple causes of disease ever compiled.* Data collected on *800 million Chinese* has given irrefutable scientific evidence that disease and death rates are definitely related to food. Even better news is evolving from computerized interpretation of the massive information: *the predictability of disease.*

By strategically positioning themselves with such forward thinking and acting pioneers as those in Africa, South America, China and India, the cumulative impact of Quantum Botanicals' multi-continental nutritional research and development can scarcely be imagined.

None of this information was available at the time I was counseling with my friend Joe James. Even if it had been, suffering the excruciating pain from arthritis that he was and had been for so many years, it would have been of little interest to him. Because, not until we met did he have the faintest understanding of the disease -- either the cause or causes. Or even -- aside from drugs -- that there was any possibility of relief. Or the remote possibility of a cure.

But now, thanks to CM Pure™, Joe's symptoms had disappeared. He is walking freely and even plays basketball occasionally. "Better yet," he grinned a few days ago, "now I'm a man again and can make love with my wife."

The tragic irony of this scenario is that he spent a ton of money to hear a number of doctors tell him there was nothing to be done and that he'd "just have to take pain medication . . . and learn to live with it . . ."

"Can you imagine?" he said to me, "Taking those pain pills for the rest of my life . . . and getting worse and worse because of all the side effects . . ."

"I can imagine," I told him. "I hear it all the time."

"Can't something be done about that abysmal lack of knowledge? Isn't it possible to do something about it?"

"The answer is yes . . . but . . ."

The truth of the matter, Joe's medical expenses could have been greatly reduced and his suffering alleviated or entirely eliminated. Yes, but how?

*It's simply a matter of health care priorities.*

It's a matter of record that health care costs in the U.S. are up to around one trillion dollars a year. Of that horrendous figure less than 2.5% goes for prevention and an even smaller amount — a mere 0.5% — goes for health promotion; leaving  approximately 97 cents out of every health care dollar for treatment; which is about everything from basic first aid to extremely costly intensive care. Nothing is spared to treat the injured and the diseased.

*Yet, little is being done to prevent illness and disease.*

At first Joe didn't know all that, but he soon learned. He did know, for example that a week's hospitalization in his home state of Montana had run up an impressive $5,000 in hospital bills, with a comparable amount for doctors. And from that figure, he knew what he had received in return. More prescriptions for more drugs, with more side effects. But no real relief for his arthritis.

Had anyone bothered to tell Joe that his suffering was in any way related to his eating habits? Not really.

Yet, it's true. What we eat has everything to do with our health.

In this entire world, is there, or are there any studies being done *on a large scale* to determine what, if anything, food, diet and lifestyle have to do with health and wellness? Or with sickness, disease and an untimely demise? Joe didn't know it, most people don't, but the answer is yes.

I have since explained the far-reaching impact of this research to others, Joe among them. "If you had known 20 years ago what you have learned in the past few months, you could have avoided all your pain and suffering . . ."

He nodded. "True. But I know it now . . . and I now know that I am fully responsible for my own health . . ."

"So, then what are you doing about it?"

"To begin with, I've eliminated all junk foods from my diet. I've thrown all sugar and white flour and prepared foods out of my house . . .

"I'm choosing fresh fruit and vegetables . . . and nuts and seeds . . ."

"What about fats and oils?"

"My wife and I have learned to read labels. We recognize and reject any product that contains any hydrogenated fats or oils." With that he sighed. "It's been difficult, but we're gradually eliminating animal fat from our diet . . ."

"What about supplements?"

"I'm taking a list as long as my arm: antioxidants -- vitamin A, C and E. The B complex . . . and so on. And the essential fatty acids . . ." Joe grinned mischievously. "Of course, there's the CM Pure™. I've got to have that." Suddenly sober Joe spoke slowly, measuring his words. "I suppose you want the bottom line?"

I nodded. "Yes, I'd like to hear it."

By way of answer, Joe stood and flexed his arms, shoulders and back, twisting and stretching. Like a Marine recruit, he dropped to the floor and quickly did a dozen push ups. Then leaped to his feet and did a score of jumping jacks. His face glowed with health. His eyes were clear. He was breathing evenly.

"This is it: *the proof.* I haven't felt this good for twenty years. And what's more. I intend to stay like this. Or improve . . ." He frowned slightly. "But, will I have to take the product all my life?"

"Would that be so bad?"

"No, not really. It would be a small price to pay for the health I have . . . for the health I have regained." His eyes held an unspoken question for me.

"I agree, Joe," I said. "I'm with you. CM Pure™ has done a lot for me, too. So much that I personally plan to take it the rest of my life. Long-term maintenance . . ."

"Every day?"

"Yes," I told him, "every day. I started out just like you did . . . just followed the directions on the bottle."

"What about now? Do you still take it?"

"Yes, I take a smaller dose every day."

"Does everybody need to do that?"

"I can't speak for others. Anyway, that's what my body needs. And it keeps me feeling good. So . . ."

He grinned boyishly. "Well, like I said . . . if that's what it takes. That's a small price to pay for good health . . ."

"Many people never have to take more than that first bottle of CM Pure™," I assured Joe. "While others, myself included, continue to take smaller amounts for maintenance, which are thought to be effective at preventing recurrance of symptoms . . ."

As I had told Joe before: Every body (and everybody) is different. So, learning what each one's body needs is each one's own responsibility. That's what it always boils down to.

Joe chose to make the necessary lifestyle changes, as have thousands of others. Their new, vibrant health testifies to the effectiveness of taking personal charge of one's health destiny.

## Chapter Nine
## THE MISSION/VISION

"Why are you doing all this?" I asked him.

"Doing what?" He appeared honestly puzzled by my question.

"This . . . Quantum Botanicals. CM Pure™ . . . all these other nutraceuticals and phytochemicals . . ."

We were seated in David Allen's spacious, book-lined office. David didn't answer me immediately, but took time to think through a careful answer. Both Barbara and I waited quietly.

"It's what I've been trained to do . . ."

"But, why are you spending all this time and money and research. There are other things you could spend your time on. Correct?"

Thoughtfully, "Yes. Yes, I suppose I could do that."

"Then, why not? It seems to me that you and Barbara are totally involved in this project . . . and you're giving 110 percent of yourselves. And, what for? Is it for money? Or, what?"

He looked at his wife. They both shook their heads. "Of course," he said, "there's money involved. But, all of our needs and more have been met, so that's not the primary reason."

"Then, what is it?"

"It's our vision, our mission. It's just something we feel that we must do."

"But, why?" I countered.

77

"First," he began, "Barbara and I aren't doing this alone. We've pulled together a team of experts and business leaders with vast experience in all aspects of manufacturing and marketing . . ."

Counting on his fingers, David named them.

"Besides Barbara, who handles the administrative aspects of the business, and myself, there's Gene Egidio, who's a world-renowned healer and author; James Turner, our attorney and Dr. B. P. Poovaiah, biochemist and expert in fatty acids . . ."

He made eye contact with Barbara. "That's it, isn't it?"

She nodded and he turned back to me. "It's a great team. Between us we have contacts all over the world."

David handed me a file folder. "It's all here, the biogs of these people. Take a look at them . . ."

The telephone rang in the next office. "Please excuse us," David said. "We've been expecting this call . . ."

When they left the room I took the opportunity to open the file. My eye was drawn to a page of quotes from leaders and celebrities. I started to bypass it and move to the file, but a couple of names caught my attention . . .

Anthony Robbins, who has advised the President of the United States, members of two royal families and a number of other prominent world figures. Tony had written, *David Allen's making a global difference on this planet . . . on a spiritual level, a health level, a financial and psychological level . . . in my opinion David is a Ghandi-like figure . . .*

. . . and Dick Gregory for another. Well known author, comedian and diet expert, Gregory said, *"David Allen is a genius, and a man of the highest integrity. Of all the people in the world who know the most about nutrition, David Allen has to be ranked in the top three . . ."*

High compliments, I thought, from men who are themselves making a difference . . .

Flipping past the testimonials, I quickly scanned the enclosed neatly-written alphabetized biogs. I knew most of these people; had spent time with some, met or spoken to the others. Impressed as I had been before, looking over this material gave me greater confidence in the vision and the mission David and Barbara had been sharing with me.

Gene Egidio, whose credentials and fame precedes him. Internationally known as a healer, Gene lectures and shares his healing energy with thousands around the world. The Russians honored him with the prestigious Cosmonaut's Medal. I also knew that this man was widely praised by doctors, TV and film stars and scores of other prominent and not-so prominent individuals for his incredible healing powers.

I took note of the title of Gene's new book, *Whose Hands Are These?* I am eager to read it.

I smiled to myself as I read the next name in the file. One wouldn't have to be involved with the health and nutrition industry very long before recognizing that name. Though I hadn't personally met him, I had spoken to *James S. Turner,* by telephone. His J.D. degree did little to describe this man's accomplishments.

And though Turner's biog was rather brief, its impact was terrific: Senior partner in the Washington, D.C. law firm, Swankin and Turner since its founding in 1973 . . . taught food and drug administrative law at the National Law Center at George Washington University.

That by itself made him invaluable to Quantum Botanicals . . .

. . . Special Counsel to the Senate Select Committee on Food, Nutrition and Health . . . member of the Food Safety Panel of the White House Conference on Food, Nutrition and Health . . .

The next one caught my eye and held it:

Advisory committee to the FDA, the Department of Energy, National Heart Institute and five food and nutrition review panels of the Congressional Office of Technology Assessment!

My head was spinning.

Those items were simply his regular law practice. The list of some of his clients included what seemed the entire food industry: Giant Food, Quaker Oats, Kraft General Foods, Dutch House, USA . . . a number of pharmaceutical companies, and his pro bono (free) work included public interest groups, such as Consumers Union, Resources for the Future, the Food Safety Council, and many others. He is also a board member of Citizens for Health.

Topping off the list: Jim Turner authored a best-selling book, *The Chemical Feast,* a critique of the Food and Drug Administration. *Qualified? Totally!*

I paused before turning to Poovaiah's pages. Dr. Poovaiah is probably one of the world's best informed persons on fatty acids, and as such is invaluable to Quantum Botanicals. His name, B. P. Poovaiah, was followed by several degrees both earned and honorary. Having spent much time with him and his writings during the research on this manuscript, I felt I knew him quite well. Officially he is Dr. Poovaiah. But his friends and colleagues address him simply as Poovaiah.

Barbara's voice broke my concentration. "Sorry it took so long." Startled, I looked up. I'd been so engrossed, I hadn't heard she and David reenter the room. Indicating the open file, David asked, "Interesting?"

I whistled. "You've built an outstanding team!"

He chuckled. "It's the best. And we're so very grateful." Referring to the telephone call, "This product is certainly generating a lot of interest . . . Okay, now where were we?"

I closed the file and put it in my brief case. I could finish it later. "Your mission . . . your vision. It appears that your entire team is vision driven and goal oriented . . .?" Unspoken question.

"Without a doubt. Their vision matches ours."

"Which leads me to this: Your mission . . . your vision. How do you define your vision?"

"Good question," David began.

"In the twenty-first century the winners will be those who stay ahead of the curve. Those who are constantly redefining their industries, creating new ideas, new markets, blazing new trails, reinventing the competitive rules, challenging the status quo . . ."

"That defines visionaries," I interrupted, "but not the vision . . ."

David nodded. He laced his hands together behind his head and leaned back. He seemed to be addressing an invisible group that only he could see.

"That's who we are," he said, "but the vision/mission is something entirely apart . . . though it must stem from the kind of people we are . . ."

"True."

"We do have a vision, one that encompasses the world. And a mission.

"Our mission is to enable people to realize *Quantum Consciousness* — to realize that all people and the entire universe is interconnected as one whole — and to empower them to work for peace, prosperity and wellness.

"We are dedicated to helping create a disease-free society and to find ways to extend our lives. Not just additional years, *but disease-free years.* Such additional years can produce additional richness so that the quality of life continues to increase with the extension of life.

"And an increase of years means an increase of meaning, of understanding and wisdom, productive value to society and prosperity for all . . ."

David Allen spoke with conviction and passion. When he finished, we all were silent, each of us moved in different ways. He spread his arms wide as though encompassing the earth.

"That's our mission *and* our vision. But, there's more," he added after pausing for a swallow of water.

"As you can see, our vision/mission is global in scope. With our combined world-wide contacts and extensive eclectic training and capabilities, our desire and plan is to comb the world for life-enhancing products and make them available to everyone, rich and poor alike . . . to do our best to produce a level playing field for all who desire good health and a prosperous life."

Driving home that afternoon, I was very thoughtful. And I asked myself again: *Who is this man, David Allen?*

Whatever else, David is no ivory tower scientist, I mused, keeping an eye on the merging traffic at the interchange at Interstates 5 and 805. He's spent time in the trenches. He knows what he's talking about. An expert in Chinese Herbology, Natural Healing and Biological Medicine, Allen has traveled the world in his quest, and is now sharing the previously undiscovered health and longevity secrets. Secrets that have been — until now — hidden from the eyes and bodies of the Western world.

A flashy red Porsche cut in front of me and I swerved to avoid hitting it.

. . . Without a doubt David Allen is well schooled in most aspects of health and nutrition, I thought. And he has a tremendous vision. But, does he have the personal experience and know how to blanket the world with all this nutritional information and products?

I remembered that as founder and CEO of Cernitin, America, he had guided the infant company from its founding, to sales of $58 million after only the second year of operation. No small feat.

I nodded to myself. *Yes, I believe the answer to my question is yes.*

Then the fact that he and Barbara are working on their new book, *Quantum Health,* based on the hypothesis that diets comprising a variety of quality foods of plant origin offer the most reliable nutritional means for sustaining healthy bodies, the economy and planet — for ourselves and for our children.

*Yes,* I nodded to myself again. *David Allen is a true scientist.*

In addition to the creation of CM Pure™, I learned that Allen specializes in the research and development of antioxidants, probiotic fermented foods, isotonic mineral salts and trace minerals from sea water.

David Allen's work encompasses EFAs or essential fatty acids such as evening primrose oil (EPO), crude palm oil (CPO) and CM Pure™, along with medicinal mushrooms, soy and other plant phytochemicals, edible algae, anti-aging precursors and enzyme-based products.

One would think that would be enough.

But I had seen some of his current work developing a new substance that will convert fat cells into protein, leading to a permanent treatment for obesity. He is also working with a scientist that many say is the Einstein of our time, that has developed a product that truly does help increase life span.

*"Yes!"* The force of my spoken word startled me.

David Allen is truly a man with a vision: a man who is asking and answering questions about health and life extension that have baffled the universe for centuries.

I liked the fact that David Allen also chairs the Development Advisory Board for A.C.E.R.I.S. This San

Francisco-based, non-profit organization was created to design and administrate a quality assurance (QA) program for manufacturers, distributors and marketers of dietary food supplements.

Personally, I was immensely pleased about this plan. Because I truly believe that this QA Seal of Approval will assist manufacturers of dietary supplements and their clients to comply with the ever-changing and evolving standards of the dietary supplement industry.

Perhaps even more importantly, maybe this seal of quality will help the consumer to shop and buy with confidence in the quality, consistency and purity of any product bearing the seal.

Heavy traffic engaged my full attention for a few minutes. As it eased up, I thought again of how positively and clearly David Allen had answered some of my toughest questions . . .

"David, is it realistically possible to extend one's life span beyond today's generally accepted three-score and ten? To, say, 90 or one hundred? Or beyond?"

There was no hesitation. "Yes!" he said. "Definitely!"

"More importantly," I pushed, "is it possible for one to attain that century mark in good health? Even better than the average world citizen enjoys today?"

"Yes again," he continued forcefully, "and that possibility is not 'out there' in the future. It's here now. Today. It is presently nutritionally possible for the person of average means to free himself or herself from the destructive forces of pain and disease and to live several decades beyond the 'age-limit' barrier society has set for itself . . ."

Driving past Mission Bay, a red-gold sun framed by a silver-lined cloud formation promising a lovely sunset caught my attention. An omen? Harbinger?

Perhaps. I only knew I had been energized by what I had seen and heard.

And challenged.

If what David believes and stands for is true . . . and it if is possible to extend one's life decades longer than the currently considered "norm" . . . and in doing so free oneself from the burden of debilitating pain and disease . . . then someone needs to take this message to the world.

Long before I had turned off the freeway onto the side street that led to my home, I had made the determination to do just that . . .

## Chapter Ten
## TESTIMONIALS OF SATISFIED USERS

From the literally thousands of enthusiastic unsolicited letters and phone reports received from grateful CM Pure™ consumers, we have selected a few to help illustrate the many benefits of the product. As you can see, these come from all walks of life and many different occupations and professions, yet report results that are consistently the same. All praise the product kthat has changed their lives.

### *Lower back pain gone*
*I used to fly fighter planes for the Air Force, so you you can see I used to be very active. But, for the last 10-12 years I've had chronic back pain so bad that I couldn't bend over, couldn't mow the lawn. I love to golf, but couldn't carry my clubs. I had to ride in a golf cart. My fingers were so stiff, I couldn't make a fist. A CAT scan indicated I had a herniated disc, and it would require surgery. I suggested we get a second opinion, so we had an MRI taken, and they discovered that my problem wasn't a herniated disc, but a pinched nerve. I asked what the solution was for that, the doctor said, surgery or pain pills, and things like that. So, that's what I've been doing for the past 10-12 years. That is, until my son told me about* CM Pure™.

*After the fifth day on the program, the pain in my lower back completely left. It's gone completely! I go out and walk the golf course. I cut the grass. I bend over and pull weeds in the yard. My mother and sister both have arthritis, so I sent them both a bottle. Now, they're both doing great,* and are able to be out working in the yard. It's simply amazing what this product can do. It's turned my whole life around.     *J.R.*

## Fantastic product!

For the last couple of years I've had pain in my shoulders, arms, elbows and knees, all of which was affecting my exercises quite a bit. Joe, a friend of mine introduced me to CM Pure™ in April and I started taking it. After 7 days the pain ceased, and since finishing the bottle in 24 days, the pain hasn't returned. I can do my exercises 7 days a week with no problems and other things I used to have difficulty with. Taking CM Pure™ has really given me a lot of good sleep and exercise and a lot better health. I think it's a fantastic product and anyone with arthritis pain or problems should use it. *D.S.*

### *33 years of pain gone!*

*During my youth and early adulthood, I was active in all major sports activities, sustaining numerous injuries to my joints, especially hips, knees, ankles and lower back. As a result I have suffered with osteoarthritic pain for the past 33 years. Just 4 months ago I was bedridden and racked with pain, requiring my wife's assistance to help me out of bed, unable to function or sleep without medication. My wife introduced me to CM Pure™, which I ordered and began using, according to directions. After only one week, nearly all the pain was gone and I was improving physically and emotionally. Just two weeks after completing the plan I was able to walk 3-4 miles a day as a door-to-door salesman without pain! Every day I feel stronger and now I am happily bringing my weight down because of my increased activities. Thank you CM Pure™. B.M.*

## Great life-changing opportunity

Two months ago when I heard about CM Pure™, I've got to tell you I was a little skeptical. But, since my family has a history of arthritis I figured I didn't have anything to lose, so I decided to use my brother as a guinea pig. He has arthritis in his knees and it takes him 20 minutes to get out of bed. Within two weeks amazing things happened to him. He could get out of bed without pain. So I said, We've got something here.

My partner's sister has been suffering with arthritis for the last 20 years. She couldn't sit through a movie and couldn't sleep the whole night in bed without tossing and turning. She got on CM Pure™ and within a 30-day period her arthritis was gone. I heard that CM Pure™ could even help prevent arthritis, so I decided to try it myself. I was having a little bit of trouble getting up in the morning, nothing really severe, but I got on CM Pure™. It's dynamite! I feel so limber and loose when I play golf. I hit the ball farther than ever. Now I'm starting to win. What's more exciting about all this is that all the people I got on CM Pure™ were people that I personally knew. CM Pure™ works great.  *C.G.*

### *This is an absolute miracle!*

*In 1948 when I was 11 years old I ran out in front of a highway patrolman who was chasing a drunk driver, clocked at over 75 miles an hour. The impact knocked me 16 feet in the air. I went over the top of the car, landed on the hood of the patrol car, up over the top and splattered on the pavement behind. The accident broke 64 bones in my face and tore my leg off below my knee. My leg was one of the first limbs in medical history to be sewn back on successfully.*

*I was in a coma for 7 days and nights. All in all I had 17 major and 11 minor surgeries. When they were finished with me, there were 1,586 stitches on the outside of my leg, 2 steel plates and 6 silver screws. Since the accident I've had pain in that ankle, knee and back. So you can see I know a little bit about pain, which I've had ever since that day. I am 60 years old now, and as the years go by the pain continues to get worse, till it's unbearable because of the arthritis in that ankle, knee and back. Over the years I've tried everything: cortisone shots directly into the bone, gold shots, the brass bracelets, all types of anti-inflammatory medications, feldane, the works. I've tried them all. They all worked for a short period of time, but the pain always came back.*

*Back in February I got a call from Bill who told me he had a product I just had to try. One that stops arthritis pain in 30 days. I told Bill it wouldn't work for me. He persisted. He said it was true and asked me to get started on it. So I tried it. I got started on CM Pure™, in within 30 days I was completely free of the pain in my ankle, knee and back.*

*For the past 2 years I hadn't slept all night in bed. I always ended up on the floor, which was the only place I could get relief from the pain in my back. But now I'm back sleeping in bed with no pain whatsoever. I'm walking a mile and a half every morning. In fact, I run the last quarter mile. I know that may not sound like much to most people, but I haven't run since I was 25 years of age. So it's just been wonderful, and an absolute miracle, this* CM Pure™. *D.S.*

### Now I can play golf again.

Most people know that if you play a contact sport you're going to get hurt, and that it's going to haunt you in your later years. Well, mine caught up to me about 6 years ago. It got so bad that both of my knees were hurting really bad. I loved to play golf, but couldn't play anymore and had to quit. A year later I had to quit dancing, which my wife loves. It got to the point I had to have a cane next to my bed in order to get up in the middle of the night. One morning I ran across the CM Pure™ ad that told how to get rid of arthritis pain forever.

That tickled my fancy, so I called the number in the ad and got CM Pure™. About the 3rd or 4th week after taking CM Pure™ I was feeling about 50% better. The

90

longer I took it the better I felt and was getting more and more mobile, even able to go up the steps without a lot of pain and using the cane.

By the 5th week I was feeling great. I felt so good that I took my wife dancing at the Elks. We did the country western, no problem. Then I went to the driving range and began hitting the ball. Now I'm playing golf. Thanks to that ad for CM Pure™, I'm mobile now. Besides that, I'm telling a lot of people out there about CM Pure™.          *J.R.*

### *Migraine headaches gone.*

*Since 1990 I was treated for sinus problems, and lately for migraine headaches, to the point that my body became immune to Tylenol, Motrin and other such drugs. I went through this for 7 years. In December several people told me how they had taken* CM Pure™ *and how it had helped their arthritis.*

*Suddenly it came to me, all the symptoms they were talking about were the ones that I had. It was a shock to realize that I had arthritis. So I ordered* CM Pure™ *and took it. After 7 days I felt something different, a healing in my head, and within one month all of my symptoms disappeared. All the pain and headaches. Since that day I haven't taken one pain pill and I have no pain, and no symptoms at all in my entire body.*          *B.L.*

### My sugar and blood pressure are normal.

I was on insulin and had chronic arthritis and hypertension. At one point I was taking 15 different medications. A friend of mine came to me with CM Pure™ and I started taking it. Within 15 days I began getting relief in my joints, so I started moving around a little bit. Now I have no more arthritis symptoms. For the past 10 or 11 months I haven't taken any of the medications the doctor prescribed for me, yet when I went back to him for a checkup he told me everything is normal. He was surprised, but I

91

didn't tell him what I was doing. My sugar and blood pressure are normal, and I have no symptoms of arthritis R.H.

### I can walk without a walker.

*About 3 months ago I had extreme pain in my left leg and lower back. Doctors gave me shots for my left knee and prescribed Motrin. But nothing helped. It became so bad that I started using a walker and a wheelchair. But nothing really helped until I took* CM Pure™. *Two weeks after I started taking* CM Pure™ *I started feeling better. Today I am feeling really, really better. I can walk without a walker and am absolutely pain free.* Mrs. E.D.

### No more need for Motrin

I have taken CM Pure™ for the past thirty days. Now I have no need to take Motrin every 4 hours as I used to. I am pain-free for the first time in over two years and carpal tunnel syndrome is not bothering me. Thanks very much. B.S.

### Knee and legs arthritis pain gone

*I listen to the Radio Talk Show, Front Page, hosted by Carl Nelson on KLJH in the early A.M. One morning Carl had a guest on who was talking about arthritis and how people with arthritis could get help. He said they would be having a lecture on arthritis as well as a product for arthritis at a place called Good Life. I went, heard the lecture, bought* CM Pure™ *and started taking it the next day, which was Sunday morning. By Sunday evening I was feeling better. At first I felt that maybe I was psyched out and my knees and legs would start hurting again. But I have not had aching knees and legs since I started taking* CM Pure™. *Before taking* CM Pure™ *my knees and legs would ache like a toothache. At night they were so painful until I would saturate them with Mineral Ice and sleep with a heating pad on them all night. One of my friends is an R.N. who has had knee replacement surgery, uses a walking cane and a lift chair, and is in constant pain. I told her about my experience with* CM Pure™, *so she ordered it, threatening me with dire consequences if it did not work. But now she, too, is free of pain, no longer using the walking cane, and of course is very happy about it. All of my friends see how good I am feeling and getting around. Yes, I am a very satisfied customer.  B. J. A.*

### Regains joint movement and flexibility

From the age of 13 to 25 of my life I was an intense martial artist. At age 35 I lost movement and flexibility in my joints, most notably my knees, concluded to be a form of arthritis, caused by overworking my joints. This related to what I was told at the age of 14 when I tried to play the bass violin, but couldn't because I was suffering from the early stages of arthritis. So, the bottom line is that I have had arthritis for a very long time. It was such a relief to get CM Pure™. After one week of taking CM Pure™, I regained movement in my knees and hips without the pain, and in the two months since, there has been no more pain. Only thirty days and the pain was gone!     *M.N.*

### *No more symptoms of asthma*

*I have had severe chronic asthma all my life. As a result I have had many respiratory arrests and been admitted to hospital emergency rooms more times than I can remember. Up until I was 23 I took prescription medications, including Slobid, Preventall Inhaler and solution, Intal and Asthmacourt for asthma every day, which did nothing to cure the asthma. The inhaler never left my hand day or night and the prescription medications left me with many uncomfortable side effects.*

*I heard of* CM Pure™. *I was skeptical, but I got it and took the capsules as directed for two weeks. After taking just the first four capsules I felt better. As the treatment progressed, the symptoms of the asthma lessened to the point that I no longer have to take any of the former medications nor use my inhaler. From the end of the first two weeks to the*

93

*present, I have had no symptoms of asthma. I consider myself cured of this affliction. Thank you folks!*     C.W.

## Reduction of swelling and pain relief

I had rheumatoid and psoriatic arthritis so bad that my hands were deformed and my knees barely mobile. I was also suffering from debilitating pain. My doctor tried several unsuccessful treatments and I was facing others that had some very serious side effects. I completed my course of taking CM Pure™ on October 31, 1996. Within twenty-four hours after taking the first capsules, I noticed reduction of swelling and pain relief. By the end of the second day I noticed increased mobility as well. I continued to be well, having only some occasional pain, which I was told was "breakthrough pain." After that time I began improving steadily, getting better and better. My hands look normal now and I feel very good. My pain is gone. Thank you! *J.L.*

### Now I can stand up

*I've had arthritis for six or seven years. I can't describe for you the pain I had in my fingers, my wrists and my shoulder. It really worried me. It worried me because I was getting crippled, and arthritis killed my father. He was so badly deformed from arthritis that they buried him in a closed casket. Anyway, I followed the directions on* CM Pure™ *bottle and on the 11th day I took it I was feeling so good that I couldn't believe it. I looked at my hands. I was amazed. I could make a fist. Then I got in the pool and I could swim. I didn't have to paddle around anymore. I could swim. You just can't believe how excited I am. I used to get down on the floor and couldn't get up. I just could not get up. I had to crawl over to a wall or table and climb up. Now, it's just, yip, and I'm up. Just like that. You just can't believe how excited I am. No pain. I could play a piano right now. I mean it's un-be-liev-able what that product's done for me!*     *N.D.*

### New lease on life from juvenile rheumatoid arthritis

When he was one year old, my 7-year-old son was diagnosed with juvenile rheumatoid arthritis. He would wake up screaming with pain. From then till he was 3 the doctor prescribed 6 adult aspirins daily. He seemed to be ignoring me when I spoke to him, because I had to speak louder and louder to get his attention. I took him for a hearing test. The long-term use of aspirin had caused a 40% hearing loss. Aspirin was discontinued and he was given liquid Naprosyn for the next four years. I knew the Naprosyn was a powerful drug, so I gradually reduced the doses till it was as low as possible. Not till he was 7, did we learn about CM Pure™ from our chiropractor. We obtained the product and he began taking it the day after Thanksgiving in 1996. In one month all the RA symptoms left and have never returned. Now, we have a normal, active boy. He's out there playing basketball like a maniac. We are so grateful, because CM Pure™ has truly given our son a new lease on life. *K.R.*

### Most incredible opportunity!

*This is the most incredible product I've personally ever been involved with. When you call someone and tell them how good CM Pure™ is, they're skeptical. They can't believe it's going to work at all. Then they try it. And then within anywhere from 8-15 days people have called me in tears telling me, they can't believe it, that CM Pure™ has changed their life. I tell you that when that happens it gives me goose bumps and I feel. It's simply amazing. You can't put a price tag on simply help a fellow human being. And it's just because CM Pure™ works. It works. I've just told a few people, and they told a few people, and it just keeps going. I'm just thankful to have had a chance to get involved. J.H.*

### Pain relief after eleven years!

In 1986 I was helping load bales of hay when some-thing happened to my back. When a chiropractor took an X-ray he said, "You've got trouble and I won't even touch your lower back." An orthopedic surgeon and neurosurgeon told me a vertebrae was broken in three pieces, so they fused and stabilized it. This did nothing for the pain, which has been continuous from the time of the accident. The drugs the doctors gave me did nothing for the pain. I have tried chiropractic, heat, massage, diathermy, acupuncture, acupressure, even guided imagery. Most of it helped a little for a few hours, then it was right back where it was before. My sister-in-law told me how CM Pure™ had fixed her little boy's arthritis, so I ordered some. I took the whole bottle, and haven't had to take any more. Within 3 days I knew something was happening: no side effects, no discomfort, nothing . . . except that the pain was easing up. I wondered, Is this too good to be true? That was in June. Now, instead of the pain being at a 9 to 10 level, *like it's been for years, now it's down to a zero or a one.* CM Pure™ is really great! R.O.

### New lease on life.

*As a result of trauma from weight lifting, I developed osteoarthritis in my hips, shoulders and neck seven years ago, along with gout, high blood pressure and insulin dependent diabetes. Despite 15 different medications I was in constant pain, had to crawl to the bathroom, and needed assistance to get dressed. This put a serious strain on my family life. I took one bottle of CM Pure™ in October of 1996. Within 3 weeks I noticed a difference. After 4 weeks, my arthritis was relieved 100%; all my medical problems and blood pressure became normal. Since then I have not required any medications for my health problems, including daily insulin! At age 48 I am now able to play with my 2 kids and have resumed my martial arts and weight lifting. Thanks to CM Pure™ I have been given a new lease on life. R.H.*

# APPENDIX
## The Inflammatory Response

The process of inflammation is highly complex and is defined as the body's reaction to physical, chemical or biological injury, which — in a normal individual — results in the localization, regeneration or repair of damaged tissue.

Inflammatory response is, unfortunately, not always beneficial to the individual. In certain circumstances the process itself can cause damage and injury. The auto-immune (which is the body turning on itself as an enemy) disease, rheumatoid arthritis, and the hypersensitive states which lead to asthma and anaphylactic shock, are examples of uncontrolled inflammatory responses.

Initiation and control of that inflammatory process is complex and governed by an array of biochemical mechanisms. One important pro-inflammatory mechanism is closely associated with cell-membrane bound arachidonic acid, which in turn, is converted into potent inflammation supported products. This comes by two pathways:

(1) The 5-lipoxygenase pathway leading to the formation of leukotrienes, and (2) the cyclooxygenase pathway which leads to the formation of prostaglandins and thromboxanes.

Many of the products of these pathways have potent inflammation-supporting properties. For instance, LTB4 is a potent chemotactic agent capable of attracting large numbers of leukocytes (white blood cells) to the site of injury. The blood and synovial fluid of persons with rheumatoid arthritis (RA) contain higher levels of LTB4 than normal. On the

97

other hand, LCT4, LTD4 and LTE4, which are metabolites of LTD4, are potent bronchoconstrictor agents and were formerly identified as SRS-A (slow reacting substances of anaphylaxis), a key factor in anaphylactic shock.

Currently used nonsteroidal anti-inflammatory drugs (NSAIDs) function mainly by inhibiting the cyclooxygenase pathway. Of course, NSAIDs may have adverse effects on the gastrointestinal, hepatic, renal, pulmonary and platelet aggregation systems in susceptible persons. NSAIDs are among the most widely prescribed agents in the United States. In view of the important functions of the inflammatory process ascribed to the lipoxygenase pathway, there has been considerable effort to develop inhibitors which block both pathways. The lipoxygenase pathway is demonstrated below.

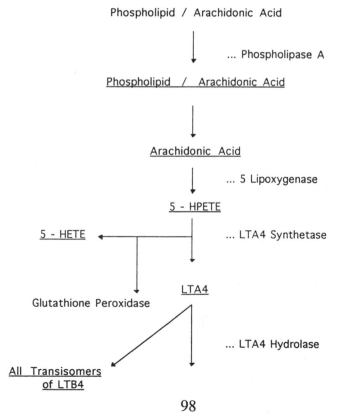

Phospholipid / Arachidonic Acid

↓ ... Phospholipase A

Phospholipid / Arachidonic Acid

↓

Arachidonic Acid

↓ ... 5 Lipoxygenase

5 - HPETE

5 - HETE ← ... LTA4 Synthetase

Glutathione Peroxidase

LTA4

... LTA4 Hydrolase

All Transisomers of LTB4

*CM Pure™ is the most potent fatty acid ever discovered in blocking metabolic pathways responsible for inflammation in the body.* Benefits are mediated through inhibition of the 5-lipoxygenase pathway which decreases leucotriene production, and the cycolooxygenase pathway which decreases production of the 2 series prostaglandins (PGs). CM Pure™ also leads to the production of the 1 series PGs (good prostaglandins that help reduce pain, tenderness and stiffness).

## Recommended Uses for CM Pure™

Because of its proven inflammation inhibiting benefits, CM Pure™ is being recommended for use in the following conditions:

- All inflammatory conditions in general
- Rheumatoid arthritis and other autoimmune conditions
- Osteoarthritis
- Viral-induced arthritis, such as Ross River Fever
- Traumatic joint injury, e.g., sports injuries
- Asthma (as noted above, CM Pure™ is a potent inhibitor of the 5-lipo oxygenase pathway which produces the powerful broncho-constricting agents LTC4, LTD4 and LTE4)
- Tissue damage and inflammation associated with many chemotherapeutic agents used in the treatment of some cancers and as an alternative to cortisone.

# GLOSSARY

**Amino acids**    A group of nitrogen-containing chemical compounds which form the basic structural units of proteins.

**Antibody**   Protein manufactured by the body which binds to antigens to neutralize, inhibit or destroy them.

**Antigen**    Any substance or microorganism that, when introduced into the body, causes the formation of antibodies against.

**Arachidonic acid (AA):** The main food culprit when it comes to producing inflammation. Originating almost entirely in animal products and saturated fats, it is a precursor to the "bad" kind of prostaglandins that produce platelet stickiness, hardening of the arteries, heart disease and strokes, as well as inflammation. Meat, poultry, dairy products (especially those containing saturated fats) and egg yolks all contain arachidonic acid.

**Atherosclerosis**    A process in which fatty substances (cholesterol and triglycerides) are deposited in the walls of medium to large arteries, eventually leading to blockage of the artery.

**Antioxidant**    Compounds such as carotenoids, vitamin C, vitamin E and selenium that prevent free radical damage to the body.

**Anti-inflammatory**   An agent that counteracts or suppresses the inflammatory process.

**Arthritis**    A group of diseases whose common threads are that they can cause pain, heat, inflammation and limited movement of joints and surrounding tissue.

**Articular cartilage**   The spongy, slick material that covers bone ends where they meet in a joint.

**Autoimmune**   A process in which antibodies develop against the body's own tissues.

**Bioflavonoids**   A group of substances found in virtually all plant foods that is essential to the health of the capillary walls, as well as for the metabolism of vitamin C.

**Blood pressure**   The force exerted by the blood as it is pumped by the heart and presses against and attempts to stretch blood vessels.

**Cardiovascular**   Of or pertaining to the heart and blood vessels.

**Cartilage**   A gellike, rubbery tissue capping the ends of the bones that meet in a joint. An excellent shock absorber, it is made of collagen and proteoglycans and protect the bone ends from wearing against each other.

**Chronic**   Long-term or frequently recurring.

**Co-enzyme**   A necessary, non-protein component of an enzyme, usually a vitamin or mineral.

**Collagen**   A vital structural protein found in cartilage that provides a dense "netting" to contain the proteoglycans, which attract and hold water in the tissue. It also provides the cartilage with elasticity and shock-absorbing properties. Cartilage is the supporting structure for the body's cells.

**Cytokine**   Nonantibody proteins released on contact with specific antigens, which act as intercellular mediators.

**Dehydration**   Excessive loss of water from the body or tissues.

**Eicosanoids** Powerful, short-lived hormone-like compounds derived from the oxygenation of long-chain fatty esters, such as CM Pure™. They lead a fleeting existence, seconds or minutes. They achieve powerful results such as dilating blood vessels and increasing blood flow, inducing powerful muscle contractions and attracting leukocytes to sites of inflammation.

**Enzyme**     An organic catalyst which speeds chemical reactions.

**Essential fatty acids (EFAs)**     Fatty acids which the body cannot manufacture — linoleic and linolenic acids.

**Fatty acid**     The key building blocks of all fats and oils (lipids) both in our foods and in our body. Fatty acids are the key players in the construction and maintenance of all healthy cells. Examples include    linoleic, linolenic and arachidonic acid.

**Free radicals**     Highly reactive molecules that can bind to and destroy cellular compounds.

**Homeostasis**     The tendency of the body's systems to maintain internal stability through the coordinated response of its parts to any situation or stimulus tending to disturb its normal condition or function.

**Hormone**     A secretion of an endocrine gland that controls and regulates functions in other parts of the body.

**Hypertension**    High blood pressure.

**Inflammation**     The response of the body's tissues to irritation or injury, which is often characterized by heat, pain, redness and swelling.

**Leukotriene**    Biologically active compounds formed from arachidonic acid that function as regulators of allergic and inflammatory reactions.

**Metabolism**     A collective term for all the chemical processes that take place in the body.

**Mineral**     An inorganic substance such as potassium, manganese or zinc that is needed in minute amounts for proper growth and functioning of the body.

**Molecule**     The smallest complete unit of a substance that can exist independently and still retain the characteristic properties of the substance.

**Neutrophils**    The circulating white blood cells essential for phagocytosis and proteolysis in which bacteria, cellular debris and solid particles are moved and destroyed.

**NSAIDs**   These are nonsteroidal, anti-inflammatory drugs commonly used to alleviate the pain and inflammation associated with arthritis and other disease or illness.

**Phagocytosis**   The process by which certain cells engulf and dispose of microorganisms and cell debris.

**Prostaglandin**   Short-lived, hormone-like chemicals that regulate cellular activities on a moment-to-moment basis. They are products of enzyme-controlled oxidation of highly unsaturated fatty acids.

**SAD (Standard American Diet)**   Food program most consistently adopted by the majority of Americans, consisting of highly refined and processed food, basically high animal protein, high fat, high sodium, sugar and white flour.

**Saturated fat**   A fat whose carbon atoms are bonded to the maximum number of hydrogen atoms; found in animal products like meat, milk, milk products and eggs.

**Stress**   Any physical, emotional or other factor that requires a bodily response to change. Continual stress brings about widespread chemical changes which may have an adverse effect upon the health.

**Syndrome**   A group of signs and symptoms that occur together in a pattern characteristic of a particular disease or abnormal condition.

**Synovial fluid**   A lubricating fluid found inside the joint which allows for smooth joint motion.

**Vitamins**   Any group of organic compounds that the body needs for normal growth, development and metabolism. Most cannot be synthesized by the body, so must be supplied by the diet. The lack of any vitamin can cause a deficiency disease.

# REFERENCES

"Antiinflammatory Diet in Rheumatic Disease," Adam, O. *European Journal of Clinical Nutrition,* 1995.

Airola, N.D., Paavo, *There Is a Cure for Arthritis.*

Appleton, Ph.D.,Nancy, *Lick the Sugar Habit.*

Babal, K., 1995. "The Arthritis and Diet Connection," *Nutr. Science News,* September, p. 18.

Baroody, Jr., Dr., Theodore A., *Alkalize Or Die.*

Belch, JJF; Ansell, D; Madhok, R; O'Dowd, A; Sturrock, R.D. Effects of altering dietary essential fatty acids on requirements for non-steroidal anti-inflammatory drugs in patients with rheumatoid arthritis, a double blind, placebo controlled study. *Ann Rheum Dis* 1988; 47-96-104.

Belch, JJF; Maple, C. Evening primrose oil and fish oils - effect in rheumatoid arthritis. IN: Sinclair, A; Gibson, RA (eds). Essential Fatty Acids and Eicosanoids: Invited Papers from Third International Congress. Champaign, *ILL: Am Oil Chem Soc* 1992:356-360.

Batmanghelidj, M.D., F., *Your Body's Many Cries for Water.*

"Botanical Lipids." Effects in Inflammation, Immune Response and Rheumatoid Arthritis." Rothman, D., et al. *Seminars in Arthritis and Rheumatism.* October 1995.

Bradford, Robert W., Henry W. Allen, Michael L. Culbert, *Oxidology, The Study of Reactive Oxygen Toxic Species (ROTS) and Their Metabolism in Human Health and Disease.*

Bucci, Ph.D., Luke, *Pain Free.*

Calder, P.C.; Bevan S.J.; Newsholme EA. (1992). The

inhibition of T-Lymphocyte proliferation by fatty acids is via an eicosanoid-independent mechanism. *Immunology*, 75(1):108-15.

Cunnane, S.C. and L. V. Thompson, Editors, *Flaxseed in Human Nutrition.*

DeCava, M.S., LNC, Judith A., *The Real Truth About Vitamins and Antioxidants.*

DeMarco, D., Santoli, D. and Zurier, R.B. 1994. "Effects of Fatty Acids on Proliferation and Activation of Human Synovial Compartments Lymphocytes." *Journal of Leuk-. ocyte Biology*, 56(5):612-5.

Duarte, O.D., Ph.D., Alex, *Get Smart, Eat Healthy.*

*EFA Nutrition News, The*, Issue 3:1, "Studies Find Certain Plant Oils Effective Against Arthritis."

*EFA Quarterly Report, The,* Issue I:IV, "How to tell a 'Good' Fat from a 'Bad' One," Barbara Levenstein.

"Effects of High Dose Fish Oil on Rheumatoid Arthritis after Stopping Nonsteroidal Antiinflammatory Drugs." Kremer, J., M.D., *Arthritis and Rheumatism,* August, 1995.

"Effects of Modulation of Inflammatory and Immune Parameters in Patients with Rheumatic and Inflammatory Disease Receiving Dietary Supplementation of N-3 and N-6 Fatty Acids." Kremer, J., MD. *Lipids,* 1996.

Erasmus, Ph.D., Udo, *Fats that Heal - Fats that Kill.*

Hansen, T.M., Lerche, A., Kassis, V., Lorenzen and Sondergaard, J. 1983. "Treatment of Rheumatoid Arthritis with Prostaglandin E1 Precursors cis-linoleic and GLA " *Scand. J. Rheum,* 12.85.

Heimlich, Jane, *What Your Doctor Won't Tell You.*

Horrobin, D.F. Interactions between n-3 and n-6 essential fatty acids (EFAs) in the regulation of cardiovascular disorders and inflammation. *Prostaglandins Leukot Essent.Fatty Acids* 1991;44:127-131.

Horrobin, D.F. Omega-6 and omega-3 essential fatty acids in atherosclerosis. *Sem Thromb Hemostasis* 1993, 19(2):129-137.

Horrobin, D.F. Essential fatty acids, immunity and viral infections. *J Nutr Med* 1990; 1:145-151.

Horrobin, D.F. Essential fatty acids and the post-viral fatigue syndrome. IN: Jenkins, R; Mowbray, J; (eds). *Post-Viral Fatigue Syndrome*. New York, NY: John Wiley & Sons Ltd. 1991:393-404.

Jenkins, D.K., J.C. Mitchell, M.S. Manku and D.F. Horrobin. 1988. "Effects of Different Sources of Gamma-linolenic Acid on the Formation of Essential Fatty Acid and Prostanoid Metabolites." *Med. Sci. Res*. 16;525.

Johnston, P.A. 1983. Book Reviews: "Clinical Uses for Essential Fatty Acids," edited by D.F. Horrobin.In: JAOCS.60;6:1088.

Jordan, Larry, *Nutrition Notebook.*

Levanthal, L. J., Boyce, E.G. and Zurier, R.B. 1993. "Treatment of Rheumatoid Arthritis with GLA.," Annals of Internal Med., 119:867.

Melina, R.D., Vesanto, Brenda Davis, R.D., Victoria Harrison, R.D., *Becoming Vegetarian.*

Moosbrugger, I.; Bischoff, P.; Beck, J.P.; Luu, B.; Borg, J. (1992). Studies on the immunological effects of fatty alcohols. *International Journal of Immunopharmacology*. V14, No2. pp. 293-302.

Murray, N.D., Michael and Joseph Pizzorno, N.D., *Encyclopedia of Natural Medicine.*

Hunt, M.D., Douglas H*., BOOM, You're Well.*

*Health Supplement Retailer,* April 1986, "Hemp Oil Available as Healthy Source for EFAs."

*Inner Light International Product Catalog.*

McDougall, M.D., John A. McDougall's *Medicine, A Challenging Second Opinion.*

Purasiri, P.; Ashby, J.; Heys, S.D.; Eremin, O. (1994). Effect of essential fatty acids on circulating T cell subsets in patients with colorectal cancer. *Cancer Immunology, Immunotherapy*, 39(4):217-22.

Rogers, M.D., Sherry A., *The Cure Is in the Kitchen.*

Rogers, M.D., Sherry A., *Wellness Against All Odds.*

Soyland, E.; Nensefer, M.S.; Braathen, L.; Drevon, C.A. (1993). Very long chain n-3 and n-6 polyunsaturated fatty acids inhibit proliferation of human T-lymphocytes in vitro. *European Journal of Clinical Investigation*, 23(2):112-21.

San Francisco Medical Research Foundation, *The Human Ecology Program.*

Tate, G., Mandell, B.F., Laposata, D., Ohliger, D., Baker, D.G., Schumacher, H.T. and Zurier, R.B. 1989. Suppression of Acute and Chromic Inflammation by Dietary Gamma-linolenic Acid. *J. Rheumatol.* 16:729

Theodosakis, M.D., M.S., M.P.H., Jason, Brenda Adderly, M.H.A., and Barry Fox, Ph.D., *The Arthritis Cure.*

The Total EFA™, *Meets your daily Essential Fatty Acid needs.*

Vogel, Dr. H.C.A., *The Nature Doctor.*

Watson, J., Byers, M.L., Mcgill, P. and Kelman, A.W. 1993. "Cytokine and Prostaglandin Production by Monoocytes of Volunteers and Rheumatoid Arthritis Patients Treated with Black Currant Seed Oil." *Br. J. Rheum.* 333:847.

Weil, M.D. Andrew, *8 Weeks to Optimum Health.*

Williams, L.L.; Kiecolt-Glaser, J.K.; Horrocks, L.A.; Hillhouse, J.T., Glaser, R. (1992). Quantitative association between altered plasma esterified omega-6 fatty acid proportions and psychological stress. *Prostaglandins, Leukotrienes and Essential Fatty Acids,* 47(2):165-70.

Young, Ph.D., D.Sc., Robert O., *Sick & Tired, The Etiology of Human Disease.*

Zurier, R.B. (1993). Fatty acids, inflammation and immune responses. *Prostaglandins, Leukotrienes and Essential Fatty Acids,* V 48:57-62.

Zurier, R.B. 1995. " Treatment of Rheumatoid Arthritis with GLA." American Oil Chemists' Society Meeting. San Antonio, Texas.